Resistance Band Workout

Stretching Exercise and Strength Training to Lose Weight and Get a Fit and Well Defined Body at Home.

Aletha Solomon

Table of Contents

Chapter 6: Upper Body Resistance Band Exercises

Chapter 11: Eating Your Way to a Healthier Lifestyle

Portion Sizes and Servings

Counting Calories

It's Not All About the Fat

You Don't Have to Give up Sugar

Introduction

Congratulations on purchasing *Resistance Band Workout*, and thank you for doing so!

We know achieving a stronger body is the main goal for many, but we also know the road there can be complicated. There are memberships to buy, trainers to pay, and hundreds of dollars worth of equipment to invest in, all of which make it hard to feel like the results you want are achievable.

The truth is you don't need a room in your house dedicated to exercise equipment to get the body you want. Resistance bands provide a challenging but also achievable means of toning up your body without the need for overpriced equipment or gym fees.

The following chapters will discuss the wide world of resistance bands, including the kinds available to you, proper usage, and detailed exercises that will be easy to adapt into any lifestyle. It can be difficult to find workout regimens that say the word 'beginner' and mean it, but we do. We'll start at beginner and work up from there, so no matter where you are at in your fitness journey, there will be exercises that challenge you but that won't overexert you. If you're already an expert, we'll provide you with reasonably advanced exercises that will help you keep pushing yourself to achieve more.

There are plenty of books on this subject on the market, thanks again for choosing this one! Every effort was made to ensure it is full of as much useful information as possible. Please enjoy!

A special thanks to my friend **Kevin Moses** and his facebook group "**Online Resistance Band Workouts**" for being a source of inspiration. Thank you so much guys

Thanks again for choosing this book, if you like leave a short review on Amazon, I would love it.

Chapter 1: Resistance Bands for a Stronger Lifestyle

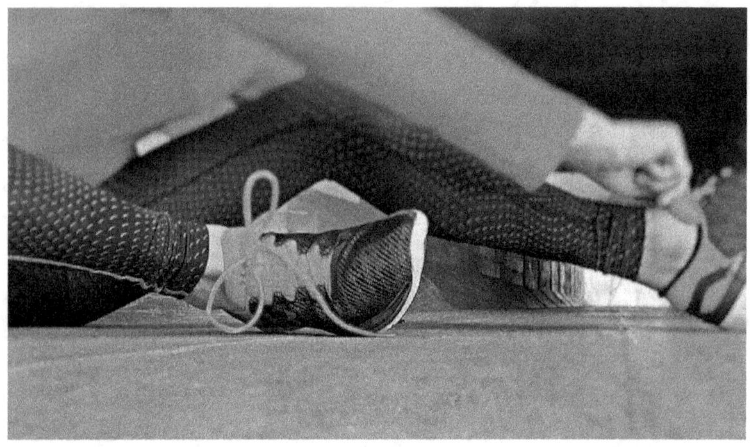

It's a little hard to believe that there's any piece of equipment under the one-hundred-dollar mark that can give your entire body a workout strong enough to build significant muscle and tone. If you're skeptical at this point, we completely get it. But we're telling you the truth, and the best part is, you can even get a full-body resistance band workout with a less than fifty dollar investment, and this book exists to show you how. So, stay tuned!

So, what's the big deal about resistance bands? They're seen hanging up in gyms and even in physical therapy establishments, but maybe you've never really seen anyone working out with them. Or maybe you have seen people working out with them online, but only with the resistance bands that are intended for glutes. "Booty bands," such as those resistance bands are commonly called, have become a recent trend in training videos, but they're far from the only option out there. That being said, let's get back to the bare basics.

What Are Resistance Bands?

A resistance band is a stretchy, elastic length of material, usually latex. Most often, this material is in the form of a firm cord or in the shape of a flat loop, somewhat like a giant rubber band.

These bands, in any shape or form, are normally assigned a weight class. This weight is not the weight of the resistance band itself if you were just holding it in your hands. Instead, the weight of the resistance band determines how much force you'll need to exert before the band will start to stretch. Weight classes typically range anywhere from 80 ounces to 2,400 ounces or more (around 2,267 to 68,038 grams, or 5 to 150 pounds). So, if it's an 80-ounce band, it will take 80 ounces of force from you to begin stretching the band. The higher the weight of the band, the more strength it will take to stretch it.

There are many different kinds of resistance bands out there, but they all follow the same basic principle. The more you stretch them, the more difficult the exercise becomes. For this reason, resistance bands are especially versatile tools. Even if you don't have a full set of resistance bands with different weights, one resistance band can provide you with a dynamic range of difficulty depending on how tight you stretch it.

Why Are Resistance Bands So Beneficial?

By now, you may already have a workout routine established, and if so, you may be wondering what more resistance bands can do for you that your current workout can't. Or maybe you haven't started working out yet, but you're wondering why you should go the resistance band route instead of doing the usual squats, crunches, or bicep curls. Let's shed some light on the many uses and benefits.

What They Can Help You With

Resistance bands aren't limited to a single capability. Unlike many exercises, which are either intended to build muscle strength or muscle endurance, but not necessarily both, resistance bands *are* well known for providing both these benefits to your body. A lighter weight band used with a bicep curl, for instance, allows you to do more repetitions of an exercise in order to build your muscle endurance, which is the ability of your muscle to do the same exercise repeatedly. Plus, the same band stretched tighter during the same exercise, or a heavier band will effectively build muscle strength, which is the amount of force your muscle can exert in one go.

Muscle strength and muscle endurance, however, are certainly not the only two benefits. Resistance bands are also extremely useful at developing:

- Muscle tone
- Flexibility
- Range of motion
- Stability

Additionally, resistance bands are commonly used in physical therapy for low-intensity muscle and joint rehabilitation after injuries or surgeries. The list of applications for either workout or recovery, either high intensity or low intensity, is astounding. This versatility has earned them a place in the workout arsenal of many trained athletes as well as the home studios (or living rooms) of fitness fanatics and fitness beginners alike.

How Resistance Bands Push You Further

Are you already on a workout routine? Way to go! Starting and keeping a workout routine are two of the hardest things we can push ourselves to accomplish, but do you feel like you could get more out of your workout? Have you stagnated or gotten bored of what you're doing? Do you want to go up to the next heaviest hand weights but can't justify what they'll cost you?

Mix things up with a set of resistance bands! Not only are they more affordable and portable than another set of dumbbells, but they are also capable of pushing you further in new ways, with a variety of exercises that will keep you interested and challenged.

Possibly one of the greatest benefits of resistance bands lies in the name. You got it—"resistance." Many other exercises force you to focus your efforts on one point of muscle contraction in order to build strength in the muscle that is being targeted. For example, a squat forces your glutes to contract as you're rising from the squatting position. With resistance bands, however, you're exercising while also working on stretching the band, which means you're constantly resisting the band's desire to return to its original shape. This forces your muscles to work at each stage of the exercise, as opposed to just one part of the exercise.

So, if you're stretching a resistance band apart horizontally with both hands, for instance, your muscles are both working on stretching it apart, and (if the exercise is done right) your muscles are also working to fight the band's pull to return to normal on your way back in.

This concept really ensures that you're getting the most out of any exercise. You'll be investing the same amount of time in an exercise you may already be doing regularly, but you'll be working your muscles in a completely new way.

For Flexibility's Sake

Let's be real. Not all of us are interested in building significant muscle. Some of us just want to tone or tighten up our bodies, and some of us just want to increase our flexibility or stretch daily while finding our most harmonious state of mind. Even for those who are interested in building muscle, stretching and flexibility are a must.

For all this, resistance bands also come in handy.

As far as stretching is concerned, some stretches, especially when mobility is limited, can be difficult to achieve. Many of us have been following along with stretching videos before that are supposed to be calming; meanwhile, those of us on the other side of the video are scratching our heads trying to figure out how an untrained person is supposed to get in that position in the first place.

With resistance bands in use, you are more easily able to control the depth of the stretch by using the band for stability. This also helps you get into great, deep stretching positions that may not have been a possibility for you before. Resistance bands can be used as an extension of yourself to easily hold your stretch in place, allowing yourself to adjust the intensity at will by gripping more or less of the band.

Take a classic sitting toe touch stretch, for example. It is common to reach for your toes with your hands and bounce closer to and further from your toes as you try to hold the stretch. One spot is too intense of a stretch to hold, and the next is not enough.

In a position like this, the hold of the stretch also relies on the ability of our hands to stay outstretched to our toes in one place and the ability of our torso to stay where the optimal part of the stretch is for us. It takes a lot of body control and focus to do both, so instead of focusing on the stretch, we are focusing on how we're going to stay in the stretch.

Now, factor in a resistance band. With the same exercise, a resistance band can be looped around the feet while the arms grip the other side. Now we have the stability and control to be able to enjoy and focus on our stretch. Increasing the intensity of the stretch is as easy as grasping the resistance band closer to the feet, and decreasing the stretch can be achieved by grasping the resistance band further away from the feet.

We'd be lying if we didn't say resistance bands are often understated or underestimated. But their ability to be used to enhance a variety of common exercises as well as introduce new ones to your routine is worth having even just one in your closet.

Given this, now it's time to pick a band, get familiar with how to use it, and get started.

Chapter 2: Common Types of Resistance Bands

If you've ever been on the internet looking for resistance bands before, you may have noticed that the variety to choose from can be a little overwhelming. Some have handles, some don't. Some sets are simple, and some come with more clips, bands, and attachments than it's possible to know what to do with.

When it comes to assessing where you are at in your fitness journey or where your mobility stands, we want to help you know what to look for in a resistance band. After all, nothing's worse than doing your shopping online and finally receiving your resistance bands only to find you can't use them for what you thought or that it's too difficult to use them. As easy as it is to make quick returns these days, we still don't want to have to send a purchase back if we can avoid it.

Let's take a deep dive into some of the more common types of resistance bands and their uses.

Power Resistance Bands (Loop Bands)

One of the most common types, power resistance bands, are also the simplest. These bands are a continuous loop and look like a giant rubber band. There are no clips or handles to worry about, and typically sets of these bands are fairly simple. Sets normally contain three to five bands of varying weights, which makes them a good choice for both the beginners and the more advanced.

For beginners, a usual set of power bands begins at a weight of around 80 ounces for the smallest band (2,267 grams / 5 pounds), although sometimes you can find sets that start a little lighter. Some of the highest bands in this category can reach around 2,400 ounces (68,038 grams / 150 pounds).

Although these bands are similar, they are not what's commonly known as "booty bands." Power resistance bands are much longer and reach a much higher weight than "booty bands" do.

Power resistance bands are also known as pull-up assistance bands. Due to their strength and length, they are sometimes secured around pull-up bars and looped around the knees during pull-ups to help support your body weight while you work on the exercise.

Like many bands, power resistance bands are also suitable for use with building muscle strength and endurance. They are also commonly used for warm-ups, stretching, and physical therapy. Thanks to their simplicity and range, these bands are some of the most versatile overall.

Tube Resistance Bands

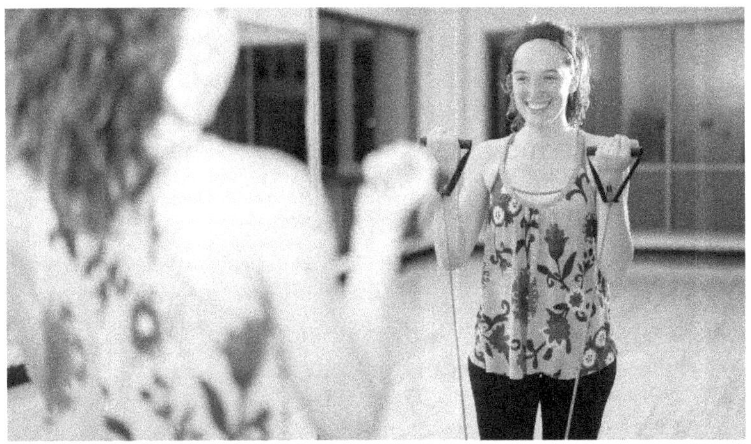

Tube resistance bands are one of the types most commonly seen in stores. These bands are made of a long cord of elastic material and typically have padded handles on either end, which makes them more friendly to those who may have difficulty holding on to a plain loop band or to those with allergies to materials in the bands.

Lighter weight tube resistance bands in a set often start at around 160 ounces (4,535 grams / 10 pounds). On the heavier side, these bands can reach around 800 ounces (22,679 grams / 50 pounds).

You don't get as much of a weight range out of these bands as you would with power resistance bands, so if you reach a point in your fitness journey where you need a higher challenge than what tube resistance bands provide, you may be looking at a different set.

For many, however, this weight range is more than suitable and will allow for a significant progressive challenge.

Tube resistance bands help with muscle strength and muscle endurance, as well as range of motion improvement and body rehabilitation. The handles make them easy to hold on to, but they may get in your way for some exercises. So when choosing tube resistance bands, it's important to take into account the types of exercises that you'd like to accomplish and if tube bands meet all your needs for those exercises without hindering you.

Mini Resistance Bands (Hip Circle Bands)

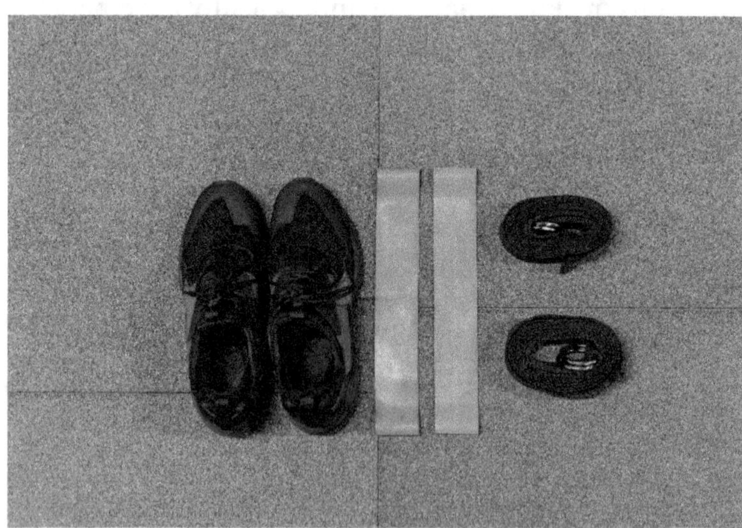

Here it is, the moment we've all been waiting for! Yes, ladies and gents, these are the bands trending on workout videos, most often referred to as the "booty band." If your main goal is to shape up those glutes, this is the go-to band. That's not to say that other resistance bands can't be paired with glute-building exercises. They certainly can. Mini bands, however, are most often used to isolate and target the glutes throughout exercises like squats, lunges, etcetera.

Mini bands are loops like power resistance bands, but they are much smaller. It's common for them to be made of fabric now with a non-slip grip inside instead of rubber latex. This is because they are intended to rest around your thighs above your knees, or sometimes around your calves just below your knees. The fabric and the non-slip backing that most of them have prevents them from rolling up on your legs or slipping down.

That being said, there are plenty of other exercises you can do with mini bands that will work your entire body, not just your glutes. While the fabric mini bands have a specialized purpose, they may also get in your way or be uncomfortable if you're intending to use them for more than just your glutes. So, there are also many other rubber mini bands on the market that are more like power bands, simple and versatile.

The lightest weight mini bands typically range around 80 ounces (2,267 grams / 5 pounds). On the heavier side, mini-bands can go as high as 800 ounces (22,679 grams / 50 pounds). These bands are sometimes also generically labeled as light, medium, and heavy weight.

We've already bolstered the booty benefits, but what else can these little power-packed bands do? Well, they are exceptional for use in strengthening your core and increasing stability. Just like with most resistance bands, they both help build muscle strength and muscle endurance (in more than just your glutes). They can easily be used for arm, shoulder, and torso-focused exercises.

If resistance bands weren't already portable enough, mini bands can fit in almost anything and be taken almost anywhere. Fabric mini bands may be slightly bulkier when folded or rolled up than rubber mini-bands are, but both can easily slip in a purse, pocket, or drawer.

Therapy Resistance Bands

Therapy resistance bands are one long and very thin band, not usually a loop (although you can tie them into one if needed). They start a lot lighter than most other bands and are normally intended for use with physical therapy and rehabilitation after injury or surgery. However, that's certainly not all they're useful for.

This type of resistance band normally averages at a weight of 48 ounces (1,360 grams / 3 pounds) on the lighter end, and the heaviest tend to have a weight of around 160 ounces (4,535 grams / 10 pounds).

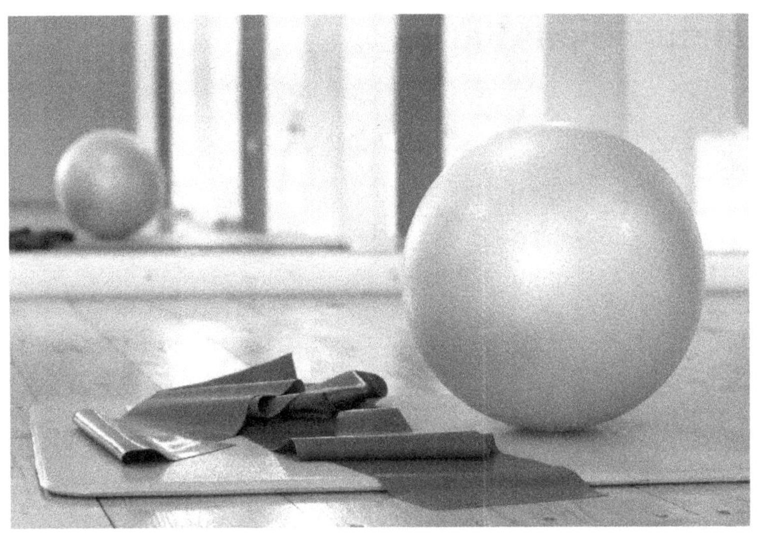

Having a lighter starting weight makes these bands especially body-friendly, which not only works well for those in physical therapy but also those who are just beginning. You can use them as-is, or you can turn them into a loop band by tying a knot in them, which opens you up to more exercise options and positions that looped bands may not always be the best at.

Not to be underestimated, therapy bands are excellent entry-level bands for building muscle strength and starting on a weight loss journey. Like the other bands, they are great tools for increasing flexibility. So if you're still unsure about resistance bands or if you're starting with limited or low strength, this is a solid place to start! Or even if you just need a simple band for pilates exercises or warm-ups, therapy bands are a reliable go-to.

Figure Eight Bands

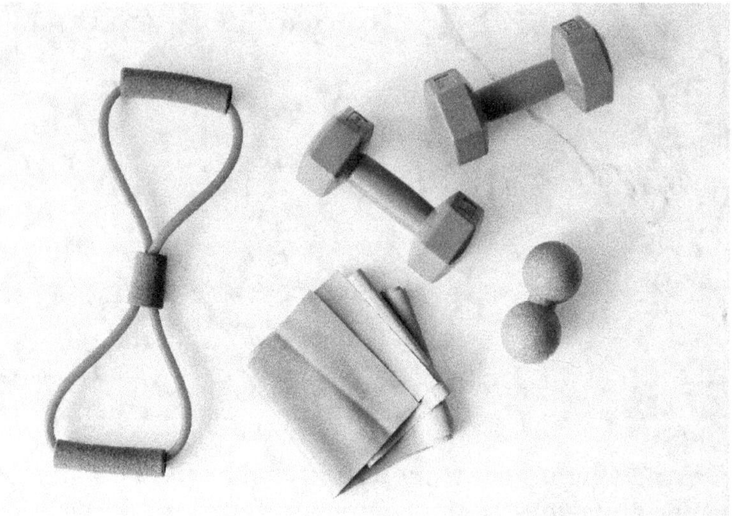

Figure eight bands live up to their name of course. Imagine a looped cord resistance band, and then clip the loop together in the middle to form the shape of an eight. There you have it! Each end of the band features a handle, and the band is short (usually about shoulder-width in length).

On average, figure eight resistance bands start around a weight of 128 ounces (3,628 grams / 8 pounds) and can go as high as 320 ounces (9,071 grams / 20 pounds).

These bands are especially helpful for exercises that involve pulling and are as exceptional as any other at building muscle strength and endurance. They offer weights that are a nice middle ground between power bands and tube bands, and their short length makes them a good choice for exercises that stay close to the body, like mini-bands. But if mini bands are more difficult or uncomfortable to hold on to, figure eight bands provide a nice cushioned grip.

Figure eight bands are typically seen used with arm exercises, but they also have applications for building strength in the legs and glutes. So if a cord resistance band is more your style, but you want something more the size of a mini-band, go for a figure eight!

Chapter 3: Maximize Results Without Injury

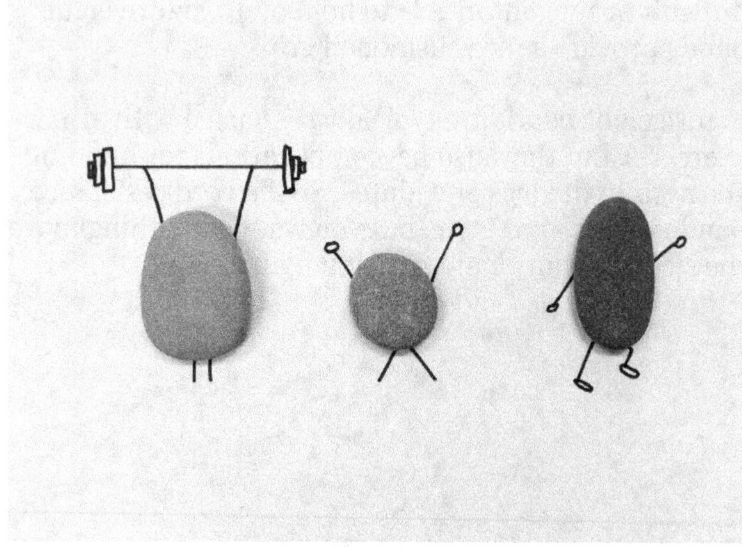

Generally, we look at resistance bands as a way to boost the gains from your exercise without putting yourself at risk of common injuries that accompany the use of some other types of heavy equipment. Resistance bands force you to take it slow while you fight the pull of the band and don't require or encourage the explosive muscle movements we sometimes see in the use of hand weights, for example. However, this doesn't mean that resistance bands can't cause injuries if used inappropriately.

We could say the same of any other exercise equipment. A good majority of exercise-related injuries are the result of improper use of the equipment or improper form while using the equipment.

Simply put, if you're not taking it slow and steady, you're doing it wrong. Resistance band exercises aren't a race, and it's important to pay attention to proper usage in order to avoid hurting yourself. No one likes an unexpected hospital visit, and the last thing you want when you've finally started an exciting new fitness routine is to be stuck on the couch with an injury for the next few weeks.

Slow Build, Slow Release

Resistance bands always want to return to their natural resting state; this is a given. As you already know, you will be fighting the force of the band when you stretch it, and you will also be fighting the band when you are returning to a resting state. Both these phases of a resistance band exercise are equally as important, so it's essential that you don't focus only on the stretching phase and then submit to a quick release. You will need to learn how to divide your strength between the stretch and the return.

Don't let the band win! To truly get the most out of each repetition, you must engage your muscles from the start to the end of it.

We know that for beginners and for those trying to rehabilitate muscle strength, this can be tough. Sometimes just stretching the band on its own is taxing. However, this doesn't mean that you should let the band drive you back to a snap release until you get strong enough to resist it.

Start with a lighter weight band, and don't exasperate all your energy trying to stretch it as far as you can before you return to the starting state. Begin small and learn the limits of your muscles. If your first handful of repetitions are too easy and you think you can stretch the band more before needing to return, then crank it up little by little until you find that you are challenged but not too tired to pull off a controlled return. You don't want to go all-out on your first try because this can result in injury and the loss of the true value of the exercise.

Slowly stretch the band a reasonable amount, to the point where you feel that your muscles are engaged and working to resist it, but not to the point where your muscles are exhausted. If you feel like your breaking point may be close, begin your slow return.

You want to try to avoid reaching the point where your arms or legs are shaking in all directions with a massive effort to resist the band. As you become stronger over time from training with your bands, you will be able to stretch the band further and further while maintaining control and stability.

Always Plan for Rests

Most exercises are comprised of sets of repetitions. What this means is that for one exercise, you repeat the main motion of that exercise a number of times (or for a certain length of time), and the total amount of repetitions of an exercise that you accomplish is considered the "set."

Between sets, there is usually a period of time allowed for a short rest. Taking this rest is as important as completing the set, even if you feel like you can go straight into your next exercise.

Most rests are between ten to thirty seconds, so they don't have to be long to be helpful. If you feel like you need a longer rest before your exercise, there's nothing wrong with that, either! You'll want to try to aim for rests no longer than two minutes in order to get the most muscle-building and endurance benefits out of your exercises.

Another essential moment of rest happens from day to day. After exercising, it's recommended to give the muscle groups you worked at least one day to recover. This is the essential time when your muscles are repairing their micro-tears that were caused by the exercise, and it's this muscle tissue repair that leads to stronger muscles in the future.

That doesn't mean you have to be completely inactive on the day you're resting your muscles. The need for post-workout rest and recovery is the main reason why most people toggle the muscle groups they work from day to day. So, if you're sore the next day from working out, you can give those muscles the chance to rest and recover and work a different muscle group.

"Feeling the Burn" is Normal, but Pain Is Not

The burn that you'll feel when working any muscle group is bound to happen. It's caused by lactic acid buildup that occurs when there's not enough oxygen to feed the muscle. It's not dangerous, but it's definitely uncomfortable, and most of us can only tolerate the burn so long before needing to give our muscles a break. The more you train your muscles, the easier it will be for you to resist giving in to the burn.

Pain, however, is different than the burn and should be treated with care and concern. If you're in pain during exercises, such as sharp stabbing pains, or aching pains in joints, listen to your body and stop the exercise immediately.

It's possible you may have caused a mild injury through overexertion or improper form, which will take time to recover from, but it's also possible that there may be a much more serious injury. The general recommendation is to speak with a doctor if you have concerns or if the pain doesn't go away over time.

The Rubber Band Effect

Part of knowing how to keep yourself injury-free when using resistance bands is understanding that they're essentially big rubber bands. If anyone has ever snapped your skin with a rubber band, you know how much that can hurt. Thankfully, the pain of a rubber band snap is brief and not serious.

Resistance bands, however, can definitely hurt you if they snap back on you. They are large tools that undergo a significant amount of tension when you're using them for exercise, and if they are let go of while under said tension, it can result in serious injury. Many eye injuries specifically have come from resistance band incidents.

The good news is that this can be avoided with proper use of the bands. Just because resistance bands are easier on our bodies doesn't mean we shouldn't respect their ability to hurt us. You always want to keep an eye on your bands and make sure you have a sturdy grip on them during your exercise.

One of the most important guidelines to keep in mind with resistance bands is that you should never suddenly release them when you're stretching them. This is why, as mentioned before, it's especially important to take your exercises slow and not expend all your energy stretching the band as far as you can, to the point where you're unable to hold onto it while bringing it slowly back in. Losing your grip on the band if your muscles give out while stretching it can cause it to lash back at you and injure you.

Additionally, some exercises require you to stand on top of a resistance band to anchor it while you pull the other side of the band with your arms. There are also exercises that have you anchor a resistance band around your foot while your foot is in motion. Here are some good general rules of thumb when doing these types of exercises to avoid accidentally releasing the band:

When Standing

- Make sure you're standing with your legs shoulder-width apart, knees slightly bent (not locked).
- Make sure you've got steady balance, with your feet planted evenly on the ground.
- Ensure that the band is resting under the middle of each foot. (Not the toe, ball, or heel).
- Finally, make sure your hand or hands are gripped in secure fists around the part of the band that they are holding, with your thumbs on the outside of the fist (don't hold your thumb inside your fist). Imagine you're holding a dumbbell and don't want to drop it.
- Wear shoes.

When the Band Is Anchored on a Foot in Motion

- It's never recommended to anchor handles of bands around your foot. Handles have a tendency to slip or roll off the foot when the band is tense. So, for these types of exercises, a loop band without handles is safest.
- Make sure the band is securely anchored around the middle of your foot, and be aware of its placement throughout the exercise.
- Make sure that the band's second anchor, whether it is a hand, thigh, or otherwise, is

secure and that the band is not anchored directly on a joint or point of weakness in your body.

- Keep your feet positioned as if they were planted on the ground at all times. Pointing your toes can encourage the band to slip.
- Wear shoes.

We know that there are exercises out there that will ask you to grab a partner and have them hold one side of the band while you pull on the other. It is never recommended to stretch a resistance band when another person is holding the other end. You may accidentally release the band, which can hurt your partner, or they may accidentally release it, which can hurt you. So unless you're working with a trained and licensed professional, it's generally advised for everyone's safety to avoid these types of exercises. Let's agree that we're all a bit better off playing tug-of-war with a rope, not a band.

Finally, never pull a resistance band directly toward your face.

Now, we don't want any of this to discourage you from using resistance bands. Every kind of exercise equipment comes with its risks. Even exercises that need no equipment come with a set of injury risks if they're done improperly. Most risks, however, are completely preventable, and knowing about them is the best way to avoid them.

Yes, Bands Can Break

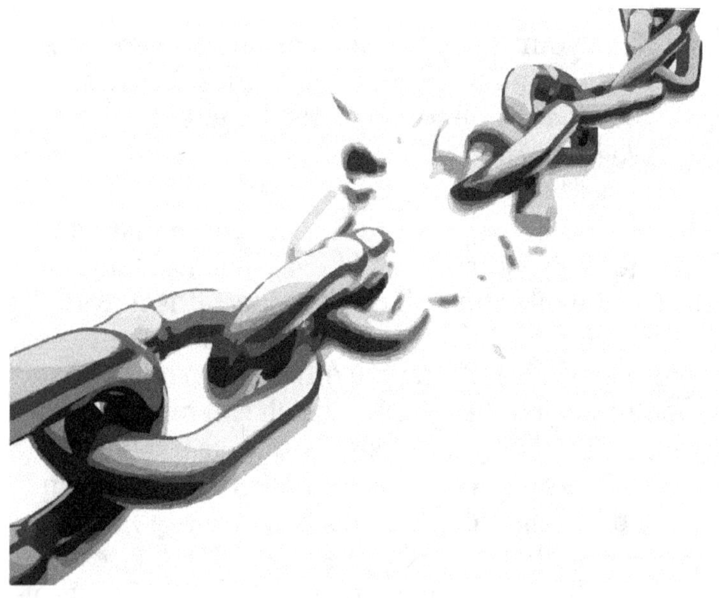

Bands breaking may be the most common concern among potential resistance band users. Just like with a rubber band, if a resistance band is stretched beyond its limits or if it's stretched at a weak spot, it can snap. We can move on with our day in a few seconds if a rubber band snaps on us at the office, but resistance bands can seriously hurt us.

For the most part, band breakages are also completely preventable. You may have noticed that rubber bands have telltale signs when they're getting ready to break, like cracks in the band or discoloration. Resistance bands have telltale signs, too, and you should always be looking for these signs any time you pick up your bands to use them.

Before using your resistance bands:

- Inspect them for cracks, punctures, or tears.
- Look for any areas of discoloration. Discoloration, where a band has grown weak, is normally lighter than the rest of the band.
- If your band has handles, thoroughly check where the handles connect to make sure there are no cracks or discolorations there. The point of handle connection is a weak spot of handled resistance bands.

Sometimes a band breaking has nothing to do with the condition before the exercise but with the way it's handled during the exercise. Like rubber bands, resistance bands *do* have a limit. Just because they are stronger and thicker than a rubber band found in the office doesn't mean they can be stretched to the ends of the earth without danger.

We should never be stretching our resistance bands past 2 to 2.5 times their original resting length. If you start to feel the band go stiff and inelastic, then it is at its limit, and you've stretched it too far, which means it's now at risk of breaking or seriously weakening. We want to stop stretching the band long before we reach this point, so keep the 2 to 2.5 times the resting length rule in mind as you're performing exercises.

Additionally, it's important to avoid jerking the band into a stretch, which is another reason why the concept of "slow and controlled" is so important. Stretching the band too suddenly can create points of weakness in the band or exploit existing weaknesses in the band.

If you're especially concerned about breakage, here are some more tips to help you prevent it:

- Select a high-quality, well-reviewed brand with a track record of providing sturdy resistance bands.
- Look for fabric bands, which won't snap on you. This may limit your options because most fabric bands are mini bands (booty bands), and most of them don't have handles. However, there are some fabric power resistance bands out there; it just takes a little more searching to find them.
- For tube resistance bands, look for ones with protective sleeves around the band, which helps contain any unintended snaps and prevents injury.

With all this in mind, there's no reason to avoid resistance bands due to the risk of them snapping. Safe, non-reckless use of resistance bands allows for an engaging workout with a very low risk of injury. Plus, due to the possibility of bands snapping, many companies have produced plenty of alternative anti-snap resistance band options. So, there's certainly a safe option out there for everyone.

Preventing Your Bands From Becoming Weak

One of the biggest causes of weakness in our resistance bands, which can be the cause of a snap, is age and heavy usage. However, another leading cause of weakness in resistance bands is the way that we treat them. This isn't limited to the way that we treat them during exercise. Proper care and storage of resistance bands play a large role in their lifespan.

No Bubble Baths Allowed

It's really tempting for us to want to douse our exercise equipment in soap or sanitizing products post-workout. After all, we're sweating on this stuff.

While we should care about keeping our resistance bands clean from workout to workout, resistance bands can't tolerate soap, chemical cleaners, or commercial sanitizers. Yup that even means no Dawn. It might be good at cleaning ducks, but it's not nearly as friendly to your resistance bands.

Soap and chemical cleaners will begin to weaken the latex of the band over time. So for these bands, the solution is a thorough water wipe-down and towel or air dry only.

Most fabric resistance bands, however, can be thrown in the washing machine on a gentle setting and air-dried. So if it is essential to you to be able to soap up your resistance bands, fabric bands are the way to go.

Don't Leave Them Outside

It's not that the bands get lonely out there without you. Resistance bands just don't do well against the elements, and leaving them outside can significantly reduce their lifespan. Imagine what happens to rubber childrens' toys when they live out in the backyard or on the patio. They don't look so pretty anymore after a good amount of sun exposure, and the same fate awaits your resistance bands if they're left out.

Both cold and heat begin to deteriorate rubber products over time. Even if your resistance bands are packed away in a shed or container outdoors when it heats up or freezes, they'll still be subject to deterioration.

You definitely want to avoid leaving them out under direct sunlight, too. If your own personal gym is outside, don't drop your resistance bands after your workout and leave them where they fell. Direct sunlight can cause the bands to crack and weaken, which makes them dangerous to use.

Or, if you take your bands with you to pilates, don't leave them in your car! A resistance band regularly exposed to heat or extreme cold inside the car is at just as much risk of snapping on you as one left outside, especially if the band is left near or under a windshield, where it could receive direct, magnified sunlight.

The best place for your resistance bands to be is in a drawer indoors or somewhere that is shaded and reasonably temperature controlled. That's the easiest and simplest way to extend the lifetime of your bands and prevent unexpected snaps.

Protect Your Environment, and Yourself

Last but not least, our final tip for using resistance bands has to do with how you use them in your home. If a band snaps or lashes back, it can cause damage to things around you, as well as yourself.

Often resistance bands will come with attachments that allow you to anchor them in a closed door. This is perfectly fine, so long as:

- Your door of choice isn't already significantly weakened, old, or previously damaged.
- You anchor the attachment so that pulling the band would only pull the door closed. For example, if your door opens into a room, you'll want to be on the outside of that door holding the resistance band with the attachment secured.
- You appropriately grip the band and don't release it when it's under tension.
- You never anchor a band, the handle of a band, or a band's door attachment to a doorknob.

No need to fear; resistance bands are here! And now that you've got all the tools you need to use them safely, you're ready to go.

Chapter 4: When Mobility Is a Concern

When working with limited mobility, it can sometimes be difficult to find exercises that are both engaging, challenging, and yet not so intense as to put you at risk of creating new injuries.

Resistance bands, however, give those with limited mobility access to more options than more difficult or potentially dangerous tools like weights can. If you are in a wheelchair or have difficulty standing for long periods of time, there are tons of resistance band exercises out there that can be achieved from a sitting position. If you have been injured in the past, or if your muscles or joints are weakened, and range of motion is low, resistance band exercises can easily be made more approachable by using a lighter band.

Being able to exercise and challenge ourselves physically is a rewarding part of our lives, but when working with limited mobility, it is also important to be familiar with your body's limits. Acknowledging when your body is not ready yet to be pushed further will help prevent injuries or help prevent you from aggravating past injuries. Becoming stronger happens with time, patience, and dedication to a regular exercise routine. It doesn't happen overnight, nor does it need to. Persistence is key!

Any Attempt to Exercise Is an Accomplishment

Your first attempts at establishing a new workout regimen with resistance bands may not be very long, or you may have difficulty completing as many repetitions as are recommended, and that is okay!

Making an effort to work toward a more active self is never easy, so the fact that you're doing it is worthy of praise. Any amount of activity is better than nothing. Over time, you'll only get stronger and be able to do more. It's not a race to get there.

Seeing exercise as a "means to an end," so to speak, doesn't always serve us well. It's great to set goals for yourself, but it's essential to constantly have new goals in mind for when you've achieved what you wanted. For example, we shouldn't aim to exercise only until we lose the amount of weight we wanted to lose.

Instead, it's better to view exercise as a "means to a happier self for life." Being active is a way of showing your appreciation and care for your body on a regular basis.

So, if you can't complete your routine yet, don't beat yourself up over it. If you miss a few days, don't worry. The most important thing is to not give up. Keep going back to it, and be proud of every extra bit of activity you are able to achieve.

Don't Push Past Pain

Pain is your body's way of telling you "enough." If you are experiencing pain that is not the natural muscle burn associated with exercise, stop the exercise and don't continue.

Give your body the time and rest it needs to recover from any pain caused by exercise, and if your pain persists, it's best to consult your doctor.

Don't Work Your Injuries

Rehabilitating lost strength and mobility caused by past healed injuries is one thing, but working current injuries is another entirely.

You should never exercise a part of your body that is injured. Forcing injured body parts to work won't help them recover faster; instead, it will make your injury more serious.

Focus on another area of your body with your exercises while you allow any injuries to heal, and don't involve any injured body parts in exercise until they are fully healed.

Modifying Your Exercises

For anyone working with limited mobility, starting with a lighter-weight physical therapy resistance band is best. Physical therapy bands are also sold in sets of varying weights, which will allow you to increase the difficulty of your exercises over time if you are able to do so.

Aside from choosing lighter resistance bands, there are a few other things you can do to modify any exercise to meet your needs.

Adjust Your Grip

The shorter the space of band that's between the two tension points, the more difficult an exercise will be. Remember, the tighter you stretch a resistance band, the more force it takes to keep stretching it.

If there is an exercise, for example, that asks you to anchor a resistance band on something and then pull it repeatedly with one of your arms, you can reduce the difficulty of this action by holding the resistance band further away from its anchoring point. The closer to the anchoring point that you hold the band, the more difficult it will be to stretch it.

Reduce Your Starting Repetitions

Most exercise routines will recommend a number of repetitions per exercise. If you're finding the amount that's recommended is too difficult to achieve right now, cut it down by a few. Focus on what's achievable! Know that no matter what level a workout routine claims to be at, everyone's beginning levels are not all the same.

It's still important to push yourself to achieve more, but do it when your body is ready for it. The more you work at what's achievable for you, the stronger and more empowered you will become. When your starting amount of repetitions becomes too easy, go on up from there.

Take Longer Rests if They're Needed

Rests during exercise are important for anyone. Take time between exercises to breathe and prepare for your next exercise. Two minutes of rest between exercises is generally the maximum recommended, but don't let this convince you that you shouldn't take longer rests if you need them. If your body is telling you it's not ready for the next exercise yet, give yourself more time to rest.

Just remember not to let your rests lead to forfeit. If you are able to continue after resting, do so! Always aim to complete your routine if you are able to. If not, aim to complete a little more of the routine the next day, and so on.

Chapter 5: Warming Up

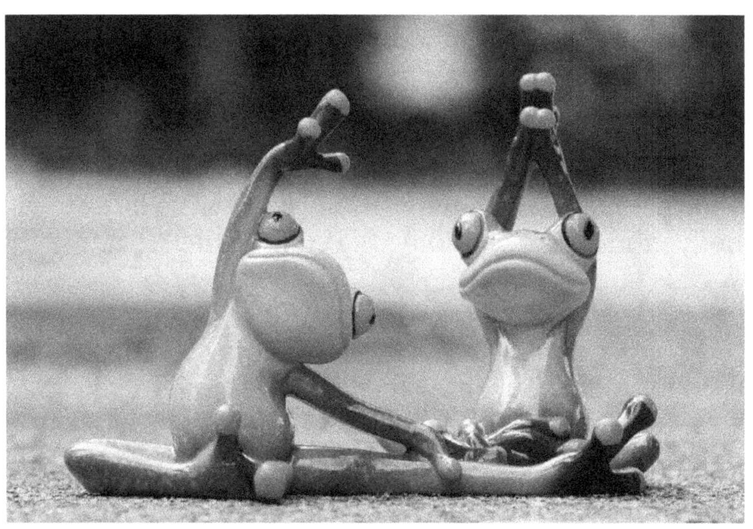

Getting down to business, there is an essential step that should always be performed before beginning exercise. Warming up your body with a few simple, easy exercises before starting your routine will help prepare your muscles and reduce the risk of injury.

So, let's get into some warm-up exercises you can do before starting your routine. Spend around five to ten minutes getting yourself warmed up and ready to go before you get into your routine!

Always remember that whether you are standing or seated, it's important to keep your back straight and remember to breathe. If you're standing, make sure you never lock your knees and start each exercise with your feet shoulder-width apart unless otherwise recommended.

Arms and Shoulders

Arm Circles (Small)

Put your arms out straight on either side of you with your palms facing down, making a 'T' with your upper body (your torso would be the stem of the 'T,' and your arms would be the top).

Now, make small circles with your arms for 20 to 30 seconds, back to front. When that's complete, reverse your direction and make circles with your arms front to back for another 20 to 30 seconds.

Shoulder Rolls

Roll your shoulders in circles from back to front. Make sure you're getting a decently sized, relaxed-paced roll, but without tensing up your shoulders. Do this for 20 to 30 seconds. Then, reverse the direction and roll your shoulders from front to back for another 20 to 30 seconds.

Arm Swings

Your arms should start relaxed at your sides. Now, repeatedly swing both arms front to back in a wide arc. You want to try to bring your arms close to shoulder level and then back down again. Do this for 10 to 20 seconds.

Next, alternate your arm swings (e.g., swing one arm back to front and one front to back.) When one arm is outstretched in front of you, the other should be outstretched behind you. Do this for another 10 to 20 seconds.

Finally, swing your arms across your front, making an 'X' across your chest, and then swing them back out to your sides. Repeat this motion for another 10 to 20 seconds.

Tricep Stretch

Bring your right elbow up, with your arm bent, and try to reach for the back of your opposite shoulder. With your left hand, gently ease your right elbow closer toward your head. Hold for 20 to 30 seconds.

Switch arms, and repeat the stretch for another 20 to 30 seconds.

Torso

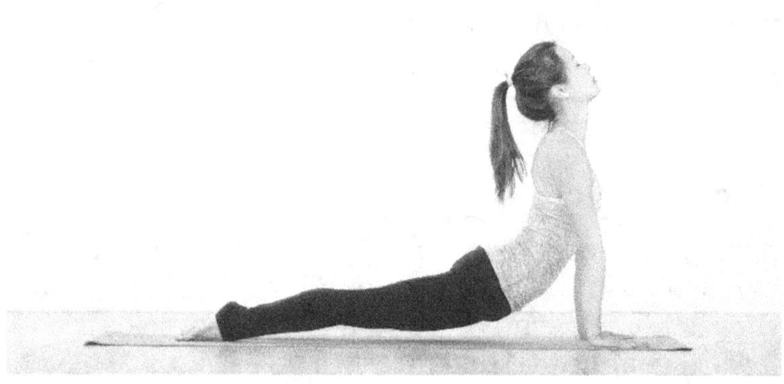

Arm Circles (Large)

This is the big brother of small arm circles and warms up both your arms and your pectorals.

Put your arms out straight on either side of you with your palms facing down, making a 'T' with your upper body. Now, make large circles with your arms, reaching to the full length of your arms when they're over your head and when they're at your sides. Start back to front and continue your circles for 20 to 30 seconds.

Slow Clap

You don't actually need to clap, but if you're feeling celebratory today, we can't stop you!

Start with your arms held out in front of you at about chest height, with both your hands' palms together. Then, move both arms back, just past each of your sides, keeping them at chest height, with your palms facing as they were when your hands were together. Repeat this motion back and forth for 20 to 30 seconds.

Star Jacks

These are fun to do and will definitely get you energized.

Start at a standing position. Extend your arms in a "V" shape over your head, and at the same time, extend your right leg out to the side as it would be if you were doing a jumping jack, touching your toe to the ground. Keep your left leg underneath you.

Next, bring your right leg back underneath you and transition into a partial crouch, bringing your arms down and in at your chest and bending your knees. You don't need to bend super low—it's not a squat. Your back should be slightly tilted forward at the hips; however, make sure that the line of your back is always straight.

Now, straighten up again, returning your arms to their "V" shape over your head. This time, extend your left leg out to the side, touching your toe to the ground. Repeat for 20 to 30 seconds.

Side Rotation Stretch

Start at a standing or seated position. Keep your arms up and bent loosely in front of you. Turn to your right to start, making sure to turn as far as you can without moving your feet (or, if seated, without shifting your bottom on the chair). Don't overdo this one; just twist as far as is comfortable for you.

Repeat this on your left next. Alternate left and right for 20 to 30 seconds.

Side Bend Stretch

Start at a standing or seated position, with your hands on your hips. Bend at the hips to your right side, then come back to the straight starting position. Now, bend at the hips to your left. Repeat, side to side, for 20 to 30 seconds.

If seated, it may be helpful to steady yourself by holding onto the chair with one or both hands for more stability.

Never bend so far that you lose your balance, and skip this warm-up if you have difficulty with balance or vertigo.

Back

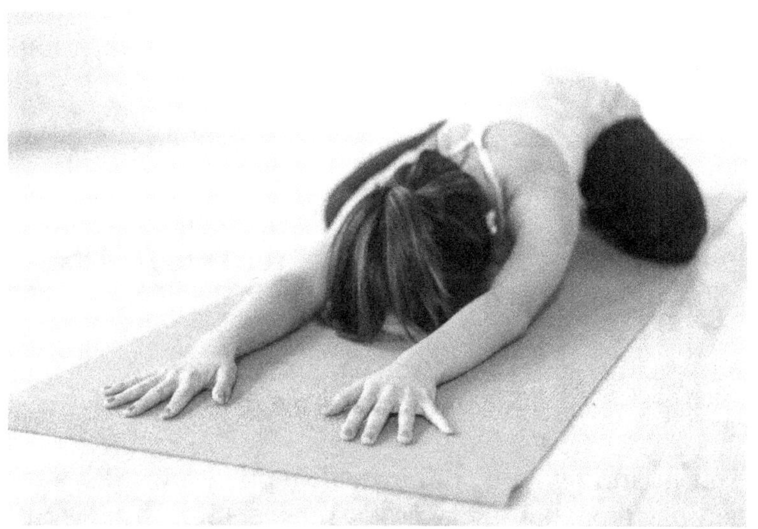

Cat/Cow

Start on your hands and knees, with your back in a neutral straight line. Now, dip your back so that it forms a slight "U" shape. You'll want to stick your bottom out to get the most out of this stretch and make sure that your head is held high. Keep your core firm and strong as you do this. This is the "cow" part of the stretch, and it simulates the curve of a cow's back from hips to shoulders. Hold this position for 10 to 20 seconds.

Next, transition to the "cat" part of the stretch by arching your back. You'll want to push through your shoulders and mid-back as if you're reaching for the ceiling with them. This form simulates a cat arching its back. Hold this position for 10 to 20 seconds.

Repeat, cat to cow, for about a minute to a minute and a half.

Toe Touches

Many of the exercises we used to do when we were kids can still be so useful to us. No one's too old for a good old-fashioned toe touch!

For starters, it's okay if you can't meet your toes. The effort to reach your toes is what we're going for here.

Start standing with your arms extended toward the ceiling. Then bend forward at the waist, pushing your weight into your heels and extending your hips backward as you do so. Reach your hands toward your toes. When you feel like you can't reach more, come back up slowly to your standing position and extend your arms toward the ceiling.

Repeat for around 20 to 30 seconds or longer.

This warm-up can also be modified for a sitting position. If seated, start with your hands extended toward the ceiling and bend forward while trying to keep your back straight, reaching for your toes as you do so, keeping your knees bent in front of you.

The Ladder Climb

Start standing or sitting with a straight back and reach for the ceiling with both arms. Starting with your right arm, reach higher for the ceiling than your starting point, moving your shoulder up and bending your spine slightly to the left in order to reach further.

Then, bring your right arm back to the neutral position, and repeat this reach with the left arm, bending your spine slightly to the right this time as you reach.

Envision yourself climbing a ladder; that's what this exercise is supposed to mimic.

Flat Trunk Twists

You'll need to start off lying flat on the floor for this one, so pick a carpeted spot, or bring out the yoga mat if you have one.

Lie down with your back flat on the floor and your arms extended out flat on either side of you, palms touching the floor.

Bend your knees and keep them together. Starting with the right side, slowly twist at your hips, bringing your knees to your right so that your right knee touches the floor. Return to your starting position, then repeat this motion on your left side. Do this for 20 to 30 seconds.

This should help warm up the lower back and help get the muscles there nice and limber.

Legs, Hips, and Glutes

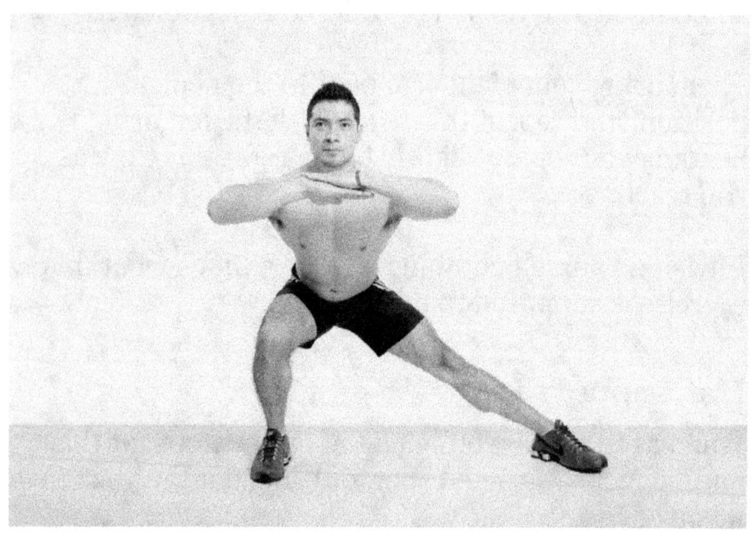

High Knees

Start at a neutral standing position with your feet together. This exercise is a lot like running in place, but we'll be trying to bring our knees higher than that.

Bring your right leg up, bent at the knee, aiming to make an "L" with your leg (or a 90-degree angle, if it's easier to think of it that way). Then, bring your right leg back down and "hop" quickly into the same position with your left leg. You'll want to go leg to leg like you're running, except you're not actually going anywhere.

While doing this, it's important not to bend your torso forward to meet your knee. Keep your core engaged and keep your back straight.

If doing this exercise at a running pace isn't achievable, no worries! You can still warm up your leg muscles by doing the same movements slowly and toggling between your legs without hopping. If you want to keep your warm-ups low-impact, this is the way to go. If needed, you can also help keep yourself steady and balanced by placing a hand against the wall as you warm up.

Hands and Knees Hip Rotations

Start on your hands and knees. Beginning with your right leg, extend your leg out behind you. Then, bend your leg at the knee as you bring it back to your side, and continue on to return your leg to its starting position.

You should be rolling your leg from the hip as you're bringing it back around to your starting position. Try to avoid jerky, trapezoidal movements. Your hip joint rotates, so that circular motion is what we're trying to do here.

Repeat this motion with your left leg. Toggle back and forth between your two legs for around 20 to 30 seconds.

Side Lunges

Start with your legs positioned just past the width of your shoulders so that your legs make a fairly wide upside-down "V." Starting on your right leg, bend your right leg as you lean toward it. You should feel the stretch occurring in the leg that is not bent, but your right leg gets a nice warm-up as well from supporting your weight.

Return to your starting position, and then bend your left leg and lean toward it. Repeat for around 20 to 30 seconds.

Forward Lunges

From a neutral standing position with your feet together, take a large step forward with your right leg. Now, bend your left leg (which should be extended behind you) so that your left shin comes as close to parallel with the floor as you are able to achieve. The ball of your foot should be on the floor, and your heel should be up off the floor. As you do this, your right leg should bend too, in front of you, and your right thigh should be parallel with the floor or as close as possible. You're essentially dropping your hips toward the floor.

Return to your neutral position by slowly straightening back up and bringing your right leg back in.

Repeat by taking a large step with your left leg. This time, your right leg will bend behind you, and your left leg will bend in front of you.

If balance is an issue, you can rest an arm on a wall to steady yourself as you lunge, but try not to use the wall, door handle, or another grip to make the action easier. Work on lunging as far as you're able for now, but don't lunge to a point where you are unable to rise.

Legs and Hips (While Seated)

Many leg warm-ups are done standing or from the floor, but plenty are also achievable from a chair! Let's look at some great warm-up modifications you can do while seated.

Ankle Roll

Sit with your back straight and your knees together. Rest your hands on your hips. Slowly pull your knees apart, rolling each foot onto its side as you do so. You don't want to move your foot across the floor as you do this. We're just rolling our ankles here, going from a foot that's flat on the floor to the side of that foot.

Roll your feet back, so they are flat again, bringing your knees back to their starting position. Repeat for 20 to 30 seconds.

Alternating Kicks

We're not actually trying to kick anything here, so no real force is needed!

Starting with a straight back and your knees in a neutral position in front of you, take your right leg from bent to straight out in front of you (or as straight as you can, no need to push for an exact straight line). Then slowly return it to the starting position. Be sure that you never lock your knee.

Do this same motion with your left leg next, and return to start again. Repeat for 20 to 30 seconds.

Alternating Leg Extension

Starting again with a straight back and your knees in a neutral position, take your right leg and stretch it out in front of you, pointing your toe so your foot is still planted on the ground while you're at full extension. Take care not to lock your knee; always keep the knee slightly bent.

Now, take your right leg back in, and swing it back underneath you if your chair allows it, with just your toe touching the ground. Return your leg to its starting position from here, and then repeat these movements for 10 to 20 seconds.

Move on to your left leg afterward, and do the same.

Seated High Knees

Here are some high knees with no impact, making them a super joint-friendly alternative to their more intense cousin, with just as much benefit.

Keep your back straight, and have your knees in a neutral position in front of you. Raise your right knee up, aiming to bring your knee almost to chest level. You can use your hands underneath your thigh to help bring your leg up; just remember not to overdo it.

Switch to your left leg now, and repeat the same motions. Do this for another 20 to 30 seconds, switching between legs.

Warmed up and ready to go now? Good! It's time to grab your resistance bands and get to it!

Chapter 6: Upper Body Resistance Band Exercises

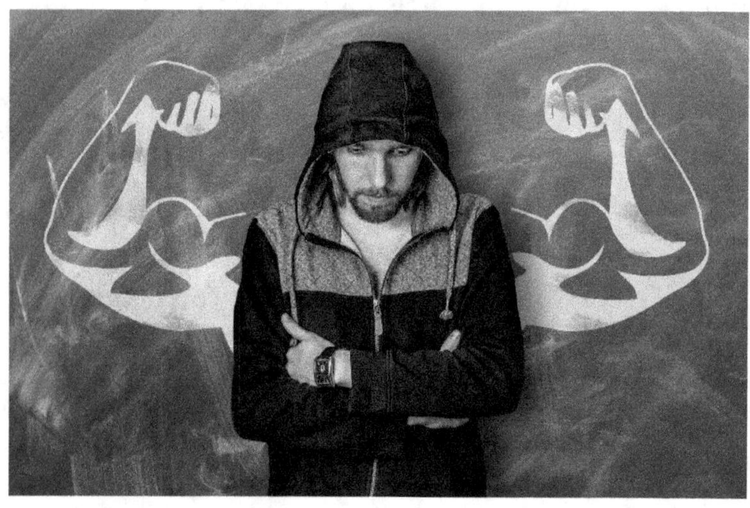

A stronger upper body can be a difficult goal to achieve; after all, your upper body contains so many moving parts! For many of us, more natural strength tends to come from the legs because our legs are required to take us everywhere we go. The upper body, however, takes more of a conscious effort divided among several muscle groups to tone and strengthen. We're certainly not getting biceps while typing at work!

Thankfully, you can strengthen every part of your upper body with just one set of resistance bands, or possibly even with just one resistance band total. There's no need to start a collection of dumbbells and then scratch your head over where to put them. Ditch that bench press in its online cart, and give these workouts a try! We think you might find them more challenging than you at first expected.

For beginners, it's always recommended to start on a lightweight band and increase the weight of the band as needed.

Arms

Pull-Apart

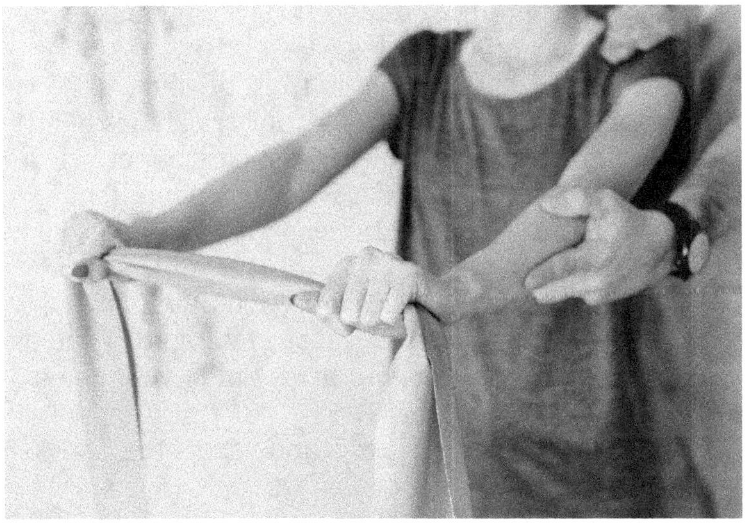

The types of resistance bands you can use for this exercise are:

- Tube Resistance Bands
- Power (Loop) Resistance Bands

- Physical Therapy Resistance Bands
- Figure Eight Resistance Bands

Beginner: Use a 48 ounce (1,360 gram / 3 pound) to an 80 ounce (2,267 gram / 5 pound) resistance band.

Advanced: Use a 160 ounce (4,535 gram / 10 pound) to a 320 ounce (9,071 gram / 20 pound) resistance band, or higher depending on your capability.

Here's the process:

1. Start standing or seated If standing, make sure your feet are shoulder-width apart.
2. Extend your arms out in front of you at shoulder height, holding your resistance band in your fists so that your arms are about shoulder-width apart. Your band should be taut at this point between your two hands but not stretched yet.
3. Pull your arms apart from each other, keeping them at shoulder height, stretching the band as you go. Try to get your arms out to your sides, so your body forms a "T."
4. Return to center slowly, and repeat this 15 times.

Bicep Curl

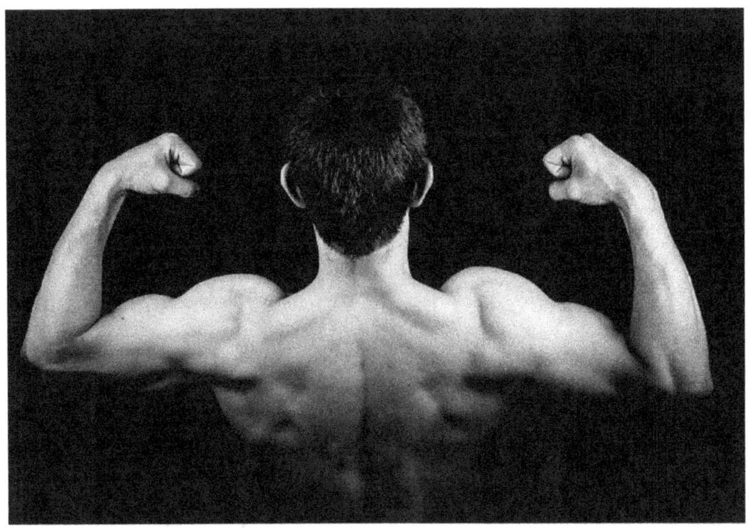

The types of resistance bands you can use for this exercise are:

- Tube Resistance Bands
- Power (Loop) Resistance Bands
- Physical Therapy Resistance Bands

Beginner: Use a 48 ounce (1,360 gram / 3 pound) to an 80 ounce (2,267 gram / 5 pound) resistance band.

Advanced: Use a 160 ounce (4,535 gram / 10 pound) to a 320 ounce (9,071 gram / 20 pound) resistance band, or higher depending on your capability.

Here's the process:

1. Start standing or seated. Secure your feet on top of your resistance band.
   a. If you're using a tube resistance band with handles, take the handles in your hands.
   b. If you're using a physical therapy band, grab the resistance band firmly near each of its ends in a fist.
   c. If you're using a power resistance band, start by holding the loop open with both hands and step on the bottom of the loop with both feet.
2. Curl your forearms up until your hands are at shoulder height, with your palms facing you.
3. Curl your forearms back down slowly.
4. Repeat this 10 to 15 times.

Overhead Press

This exercise requires a tube resistance band with handles.

Beginner: Use a 48 ounce (1,360 gram / 3 pound) to an 80 ounce (2,267 gram / 5 pound) resistance band.

Advanced: Use a 160 ounce (4,535 gram / 10 pound) to a 320 ounce (9,071 gram / 20 pound) resistance band, or higher depending on your capability.

Here's the process:

1. Start standing. Take a medium step forward with one foot (it doesn't matter which).
2. Stand on your resistance band with the foot that is extended behind you.
3. Hold the resistance band handles in both hands, and bring both arms up in an "L" shape at shoulder height (your hands should be at the level of your jaw or close).
4. Extend your arms straight up toward the ceiling, then slowly bring them back down to the "L" shape you started in.
5. Repeat this 20 times.

Bent Lift

Let's use a power (loop) resistance band for this one.

Beginner: Use a 48 ounce (1,360 gram / 3 pound) to an 80 ounce (2,267 gram / 5 pound) resistance band.

Advanced: Use a 160 ounce (4,535 gram / 10 pound) to a 320 ounce (9,071 gram / 20 pound) resistance band, or higher depending on your capability.

Here's the process:

1. Start standing. Grip your loop band with one hand over either end so that the loop is "closed."
2. Stand on top of the closed band, making sure you have an equal amount of band on each

side. There should now be an end loop you can grasp on both sides.
3. Bend forward, making sure to keep your back straight. Your body shouldn't be at a 90-degree angle here; your back should be slightly sloped up.
4. Grasp the loops like handles on either side of your feet with each hand.
5. Start with your palm facing in toward you. Then slowly lift your arms to an "L" shape at your sides, rotating your wrists as you lift so that your palms face your sides.
6. Bring your arms back down to their starting position (keep it controlled!)
7. Repeat 15 times.

Shoulders

Front Raise

The types of resistance bands you can use for this exercise are:

- Tube Resistance Bands
- Power (Loop) Resistance Bands
- Physical Therapy Resistance Bands

Beginner: Use a 48 ounce (1,360 gram / 3 pound) to an 80 ounce (2,267 gram / 5 pound) resistance band.

Advanced: Use a 160 ounce (4,535 gram / 10 pound) to a 320 ounce (9,071 gram / 20 pound) resistance band, or higher depending on your capability.

Here's the process:

1. Standing or seated, plant your feet over your resistance band and keep your back straight.
2. Take each end of the resistance band in either hand. If you're using a power resistance band, stand inside of the open loop, and grasp the other end of the loop in both fists, with your palms facing down.
3. Start. with your arms straight and your hands at your thighs.
4. Slowly lift your arms in front of you, keeping them straight. Try to come up to shoulder height.
5. Slowly return to the starting position.
6. Repeat this 15 times.

Shrug

This exercise is best done with a power (loop) resistance band. It can be achieved with a handled tube resistance band, although these bands may be a little too long when standing on them to get the full effect from this exercise.

Beginner: Use a 48 ounce (1,360 gram / 3 pound) to an 80 ounce (2,267 gram / 5 pound) resistance band.

Advanced: Use a 160 ounce (4,535 gram / 10 pound) to a 320 ounce (9,071 gram / 20 pound) resistance band, or higher depending on your capability.

Here's the process:

1. Start standing shoulder-width apart, and grab your band on either end so that the loop is "closed."
2. Stand on the "closed" band so that a loop (like a handle) is sticking out on either side of your foot. Hold each of these loops like handles, with your palms facing your sides. (Or if you're using handled tube resistance bands, stand on the middle of the band and grab the handles).
3. Now, shrug! Shrug as high as you can! Shrug like you've never shrugged before...and hold that position for a moment or two.
4. Return slowly to your starting position.
5. Repeat this 15 to 20 times.

Behind Pull-Aparts

The types of resistance bands you can use for this exercise are:

- Tube Resistance Bands
- Power (Loop) Resistance Bands
- Physical Therapy Resistance Bands
- Figure Eight Resistance Bands

Beginner: Use a 48 ounce (1,360 gram / 3 pound) to an 80 ounce (2,267 gram / 5 pound) resistance band.

Advanced: Use a 160 ounce (4,535 gram / 10 pound) to a 320 ounce (9,071 gram / 20 pound) resistance band, or higher depending on your capability.

Here's the process:

1. Standing or seated, with your back nice and straight, hold your band behind you with your arms straight. If you're using a power (loop) resistance band, hold the loop "closed" at either end in your fists.
2. Stretch the band as far as you can and breathe, breathe, breathe through it (as always).
3. Hold the furthest stretched position you can reasonably achieve for a moment and then begin a slow, controlled return to the starting position.
4. Repeat this 10 to 15 times.

Upright Row

The types of resistance bands you can use for this exercise are:

- Tube Resistance Bands
- Power (Loop) Resistance Bands

Beginner: Use a 48 ounce (1,360 gram / 3 pound) to an 80 ounce (2,267 gram / 5 pound) resistance band.

Advanced: Use a 160 ounce (4,535 gram / 10 pound) to a 320 ounce (9,071 gram / 20 pound) resistance band, or higher depending on your capability.

Here's the process:

1. Standing or seated, secure your feet over the middle of the resistance band. Hold the ends of the resistance band in your fists, palms facing down. If you're using a power (loop) resistance band, stand on the resistance band inside the open loop, and grab the other end of the loop in both fists.
2. Slowly pull the resistance band up, keeping your hands together. Try to get your hands up to your chin. Your elbows should be higher than your hands as you reach the top of the stretch.
3. Make a slow, controlled return back to the starting position.
4. This one can be a little tough, so for beginners, start by trying to do this 5 to 10 times. For more advanced users, aim for 15 to 20 times.

Chest

Supine Chest Press

The types of resistance bands you can use for this exercise are:

- Tube Resistance Bands
- Power (Loop) Resistance Bands
- Physical Therapy Resistance Bands

Beginner: Use a 48 ounce (1,360 gram / 3 pound) to an 80 ounce (2,267 gram / 5 pound) resistance band.

Advanced: Use a 160 ounce (4,535 gram / 10 pound) to a 320 ounce (9,071 gram / 20 pound) resistance band, or higher depending on your capability.

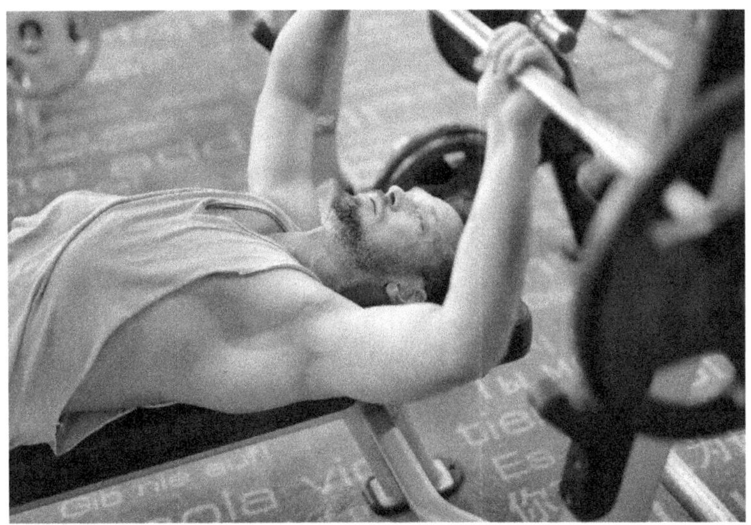

Here's the process:

1. Hold your resistance band behind your back so that it's just taut. The band should be touching your back just below your shoulder blades. If you're using a power (loop) resistance band, the loop should be "closed."
2. You'll be lying on the floor for this one, so choose a carpeted spot or a yoga mat. Come down to the ground and lay flat on your back with your knees bent and together.
3. Grab each end of the resistance band with your palms facing away from your face. For power (loop) resistance bands, you can either simply

grab both ends in your fists (keeping the loop closed), or you can grab the ends of the resistance band like handles, whichever is most comfortable and secure for you.

4. Start with your arms bent at either side of you, level with your shoulders, with your fists in the air.
5. Push your arms up toward the ceiling and bring them together while squeezing your chest.
6. Make your slow return to the starting position.
7. Repeat 10 to 15 times.

This exercise can also be done while sitting in a chair. If you're sitting, wrap the resistance band around your back, just under your shoulder blades. Start with your arms bent at shoulder height with your fists positioned forward. Push your arms out in front of you, with your palms facing away from you, and bring your arms together as you straighten them. Make sure you're squeezing your chest as you bring your arms together in front of you.

Standing Incline Press

Tube resistance bands with handles are best used for this exercise.

Beginner: Use a 48 ounce (1,360 gram / 3 pound) to an 80 ounce (2,267 gram / 5 pound) resistance band.

Advanced: Use a 160 ounce (4,535 gram / 10 pound) to a 320 ounce (9,071 gram / 20 pound) resistance band, or higher depending on your capability.

Here's the process:

1. Start standing as if you're about to begin a forward lunge, with one foot behind you and one foot in front of you.
2. Anchor the resistance band underneath your back foot and hold the handles in your fists, with your palms facing away from you.
3. Start with your arms in an "L" shape at your sides, just about at shoulder height, with your fists in the air.
4. Slowly push your arms out in front of you, straightening them as you go. Squeeze your chest to bring your arms together in front of you.
5. You want your arms to end at a slight incline to get the most out of this exercise as if you're reaching for something on a high shelf. Don't outstretch your arms over your head or straight out at chest level for this one. Aim for somewhere in between.
6. Return nice and easy to your starting position.
7. Repeat this 10 to 15 times. It can be challenging, so don't be afraid to start with fewer reps and work your way up!

Resistance Band Push-Ups

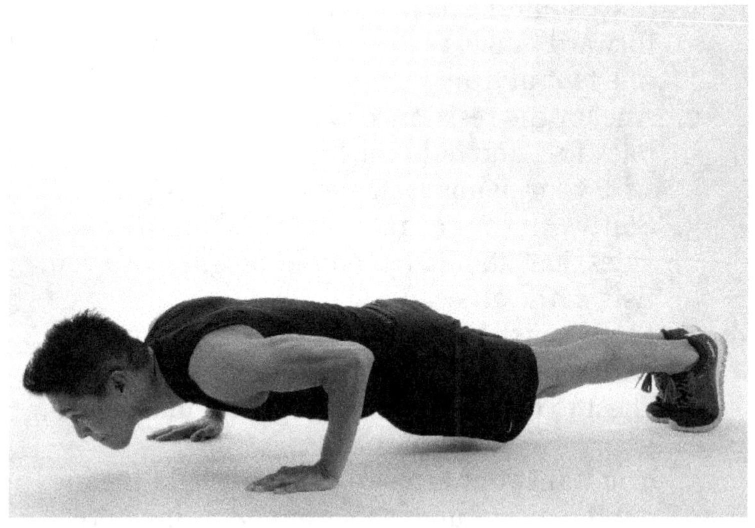

The types of resistance bands you can use for this exercise are:

- Tube Resistance Bands
- Power (Loop) Resistance Bands

This one can be exceptionally challenging for anyone unless you're used to doing multiple reps of push-ups regularly already, so for most, we recommend starting with a 48 ounce (1,360 gram / 3 pound) to an 80 ounce (2,267 gram / 5 pound) resistance band.

Here's the process:

1. You'll be on the floor for this one, and you can either do full push-ups if you are able, or you can do modified push-ups on your knees. If you're on your knees, head to a carpeted spot or a mat.
2. Get ready for a push-up position. Bring your resistance band around your back, just under your shoulder blades, and secure each end on both hands (under the palm).
3. If you're doing a full push-up, begin at a plank, with your arms outstretched underneath your shoulders and your whole body from your back to your heels, forming a straight line.
4. If you're doing a push-up from your knees, have your arms outstretched underneath your shoulders, but instead of having your legs out straight, you'll be resting on your knees with your back straight.
5. Bend your arms to bring your body down as close to the floor as you can while maintaining a straight line with your back. Don't dip your hips to the floor, and don't stick your butt up in the air, in the wise words of every gym teacher to ever exist.
6. Push yourself back up to the starting position.
7. Start off repeating this 5 to 10 times if you're inexperienced with push-ups. But if you feel like you can do more, take it to 15 or 20!

Resistance Band Rows

The types of resistance bands you can use for this exercise are:

- Tube Resistance Bands
- Power (Loop) Resistance Bands
- Physical Therapy Resistance Bands

Beginner: Use a 48 ounce (1,360 gram / 3 pound) to an 80 ounce (2,267 gram / 5 pound) resistance band.

Advanced: Use a 160 ounce (4,535 gram / 10 pound) to a 320 ounce (9,071 gram / 20 pound) resistance band, or higher depending on your capability.

Here's the process:

1. Start seated on the floor with your legs straight out in front of you. Make sure you keep a straight back during this exercise. Resist the urge to slouch!
2. Loop the resistance band around the soles of your feet and hold onto each end of the band with your arms outstretched in front of you. For a more secure anchor around your feet, longer resistance bands can be wrapped completely around the feet once first.
3. Squeeze your shoulder blades together.
4. Bring your elbows back next until they are about even with your sides and your arms both form an "L."
5. Slowly return to your starting position.

6. Repeat 15 to 20 times.

Abs

Standing Twist

The types of resistance bands you can use for this exercise are:

- Tube Resistance Bands
- Power (Loop) Resistance Bands
- Physical Therapy Resistance Bands

The target of this exercise is to work the abdominal muscles, not the arms. So, we don't want to make it an arm workout for you just to stretch the band.

For most, we recommend starting with a 48 ounce (1,360 gram / 3 pound) to an 80 ounce (2,267 gram / 5 pound) resistance band.

If this is too easy even when increasing your reps, and you feel like you wouldn't have an issue keeping a 160 ounce (4,535 gram / 10 pound) or a 320 ounce (9,071 gram / 20 pound) band stretched while you do this, then you're welcome to try it!

Here's the process:

1. Start standing on the middle of the resistance band with your feet shoulder-width apart while holding either end at your sides. For power (loop) resistance bands, stand on the band at

the bottom of its open loop and hold the top of the band with both hands.

2. Bend your arms up at your sides (like you're at the top of a bicep curl), stretching the band up with you.
3. Keeping your hips and legs as still as possible, turn just your torso to the right, then return to the center.
4. Now, turn your torso to the left, and return to the center.
5. Repeat this 10 to 15 times or more, depending on the level of difficulty or endurance you want to achieve.

Resistance Band Russian Twist

The types of resistance bands you can use for this exercise are:

- Tube Resistance Bands
- Power (Loop) Resistance Bands
- Physical Therapy Resistance Bands

Beginner: Use a 48 ounce (1,360 gram / 3 pound) to an 80 ounce (2,267 gram / 5 pound) resistance band.

Advanced: Use a 160 ounce (4,535 gram / 10 pound) to a 320 ounce (9,071 gram / 20 pound) resistance band, or higher depending on your capability.

Here's the process:

1. Start seated on the floor with your legs bent in front of you, with just your heels touching the floor. (Your soles should be facing away from you). Keep your back straight.
2. Loop your resistance band around the soles of your feet and firmly grasp the other end with both hands, keeping both hands close together. For power (loop) resistance bands, hold the loop "open" and circle one end around your feet while you hold the other end, both hands fairly close together. Alternatively, you can loop the band around your feet while "closed" and hold onto each end like a handle, but this provides more resistance and may be more challenging.
3. Keeping your back straight still, lean back slightly to about a 45-degree angle and hold that, engaging your abs. You should start to feel your abs working to keep you upright already.
4. Stretch the resistance band with you as you lean back, keeping both hands together and both arms straight out in front of you with your elbows slightly bent.
5. Now, twist your torso to the right, bringing your arms with you, stretching the band further. Come as close as you can to tapping the floor at your right side with your fists. Then return to the center.
6. Twist your torso left next, repeating the same motion of tapping the floor with your fists.

7. Repeat 5 to 15 times, depending on your capability.

For those of you that have done Russian Twists before, you know how challenging they can be even without resistance bands! This is really the next step up.

Anyone new to exercising or to ab workouts should really take it slow with this one. Try some Russian Twists without resistance bands first so you can get a feel for where you're at on your six-pack quest before amping up your muscle burn with a resistance band.

Supine Leg Press

The types of resistance bands you can use for this exercise are:

- Tube Resistance Bands
- Power (Loop) Resistance Bands

Beginner: Use a 48 ounce (1,360 gram / 3 pound) to an 80 ounce (2,267 gram / 5 pound) resistance band.

Advanced: Use a 160 ounce (4,535 gram / 10 pound) to a 320 ounce (9,071 gram / 20 pound) resistance band, or higher depending on your capability.

Here's the process:

1. Start on your back on the floor, with your knees bent up toward you. (Your legs should form an

"L." Your thighs will be up at a 90-degree angle to your body, and your calves and feet will be parallel with the floor. Your soles should be facing away from you.

2. Loop your resistance band around your feet and hold onto each end. Your arms should form an "L" here too. The part of your arm above the elbow should be parallel with and resting on the floor, and your arm should be bent at the elbow so that your hands are holding on to the resistance band over your chest.
   a. For power (loop) resistance bands, it's best to start with an "open" loop, loop one end around your feet, and hold on to the other end of the loop with both hands.
   b. For tube resistance bands, loop the band around your feet and hold on to both handles, or wrap the band around your feet once first.
3. Now that your bands secure, steadily push your feet out away from you until your legs form about a 45-degree angle (slight upward slant). Hold it for a moment, and really engage your lower abs here.
4. Return to your starting position.
5. Repeat this 10 to 15 times.

Plank Kick

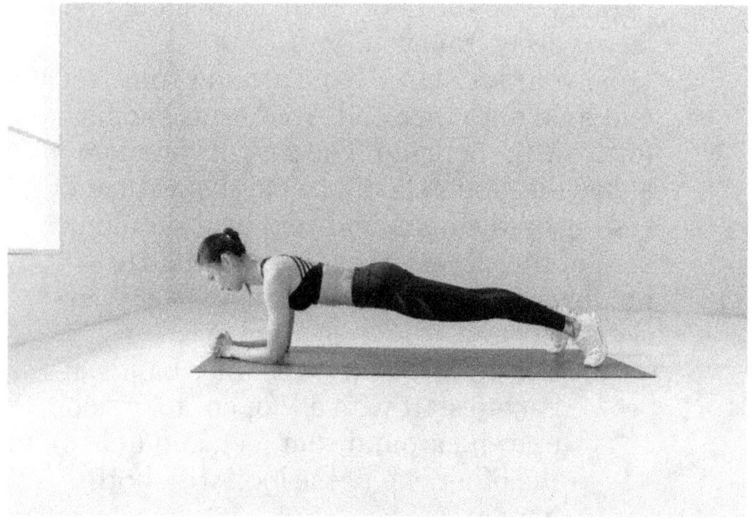

It wouldn't be a complete set of ab exercises without a plank, would it? Not to worry, your friend, the plank, has arrived, and if you're groaning right now, we get it. Planking is already tough! Add a resistance band on top of that, and you've got a real challenge.

For this exercise, you'll need a mini resistance band, also known as the "booty band!" Except…we're working more than just the booty here. Remember, this is ab-focused, so don't forget to engage those abs!

Beginner: Use an 80 ounce (2,267 gram / 5 pound) resistance band or lighter if you can find one.

Advanced: Use a 160 ounce (4,535 gram / 10 pound) to a 320 ounce (9,071 gram / 20 pound) resistance band, or weights in that range.

If your mini bands aren't assigned specific weights, start with a "light" weight resistance band. For more advanced plankers, go for a "medium" to "heavy" weight resistance band.

Here's the process:

1. You'll want to start by circling the mini-band around your thighs, just above your knees. It's extremely important to never loop a resistance band around your knees.
2. Get into a resting arm plank position. This means that your upper body is supported on your forearms, and your elbows should be directly under your shoulders. Extend your legs out behind you with the balls of your feet on the ground and your heels up. Make sure your whole body follows a nice straight descending line from your head to your heels.
3. Already tough? Get ready! Now, lift your right leg as high as you can, trying to keep your leg straight. Then slowly return to the starting plank.
4. Next, do the same with your left leg.
5. Repeat this 10 to 15 times, or don't be afraid to cut it at 5 if it's too tough.

Back

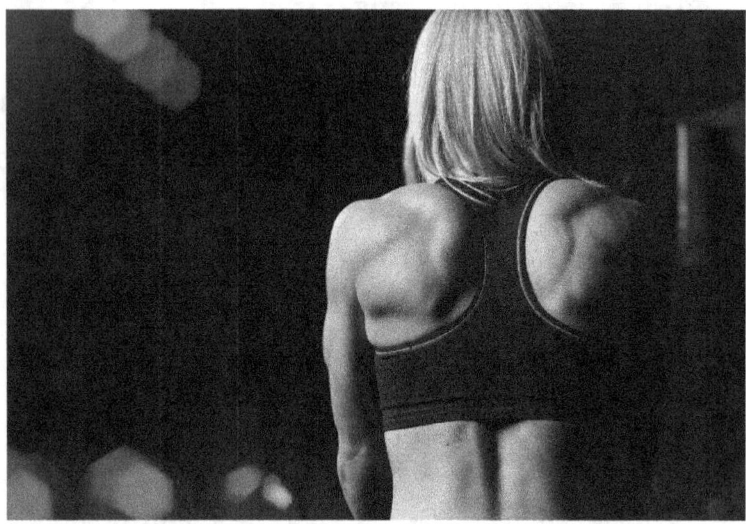

Here's a secret. Many of the exercises you've already seen in this chapter doubly work the back; the resistance band row, shrugs, and the plank kick, to name a few.

For an extra back boost, here are a couple more back-focused exercises to try.

Deadlift

Let's use a power resistance band for this one.

It's highly recommended to start with a 48 ounce (1,360 gram / 3 pound) or an 80 ounce (2,267 gram / 5 pound) resistance band, especially if you have a sensitive or weak back that needs strengthening.

For more advanced back-builders, go up to 160 ounce (4,535 gram / 10 pound), 320 ounce (9,071 gram / 20 pound) or higher if you're capable. Just remember to start light if you're not sure.

Here's the process:

1. Start standing. Hold the band with the loop "closed" and stand on top of the middle of it.
2. Bend down to grab each end of the resistance band like a handle. Keep your back straight, your arms straight, and bend your knees slightly. Make sure you are looking out in front of you, not down at your feet. (This will help prevent you from arching your back).
3. Straighten up from your hips to a normal standing position, arms coming straight to your sides. (The band will be stretched at this point).
4. Return to the bent position slowly.
5. Repeat 10 to 20 times.

Bent Back Fly

A tube resistance band is best used for this exercise.

Beginner: Use a 48 ounce (1,360 gram / 3 pound) to an 80 ounce (2,267 gram / 5 pound) resistance band.

Advanced: Use a 160 ounce (4,535 gram / 10 pound) to a 320 ounce (9,071 gram / 20 pound) resistance band, or higher depending on your capability.

Here's the process:

1. Start standing with your feet shoulder-width apart. Stand on the middle of your band.
2. Grab the handle that is on your right with your left hand, and grab the handle that is on your left with your right hand (so the band forms an "X" in front of you).
3. Bend at the waist, making sure to keep your back straight.
4. Lift both arms simultaneously, stretching the band until your arms are level with your back (parallel to the ground).
5. Slowly return to the starting position.
6. Repeat 10 to 20 times.

Phew! Now *that* was a lot of different exercises to look at and experiment with. The upper body, as we were mentioning before, is made up of so many targetable moving parts. Many exercises do benefit multiple parts of the upper body, but others need special treatment to achieve the results we want.

The lower body, thankfully, is built up of less uniquely moving parts. While it's still important to spend time identifying, isolating, and exercising the various muscle groups of our lower body, it's a little simpler to categorize them. So, let's shake a leg! It's time to get our calves and quads in the mix. The glutes, on the other hand...we'll get to that a little later.

Chapter 7: Lower Body Resistance Band Exercises

Are you enjoying my work? If you could leave a little review for me on Amazon? I would be infinitely grateful.

Many of us dream of the day that we'll have those nice strong, firm legs to show off in shorts, bathing suits, or what have you. If it weren't for all those squats, well, maybe it'd be a lot easier! The truth is, squats are far from the only challenging exercise you can do for your legs. Don't worry, squats weren't all we had planned.

Resistance bands are extremely important for leg exercises, as well. Whereas leg exercises without bands will certainly tone your legs, including a resistance band in your exercise helps to work those small muscle groups that are a big part of overall leg strength and shape but which are often hard to target and isolate otherwise.

Many exercises for the legs are best achieved with a mini resistance band. After all, the size of these bands usually provides perfect resistance when circled around the legs. There are some other exercises that are able to work the legs perfectly well with the other major types of resistance bands, and we'll include a few here, too.

Thighs and Hips

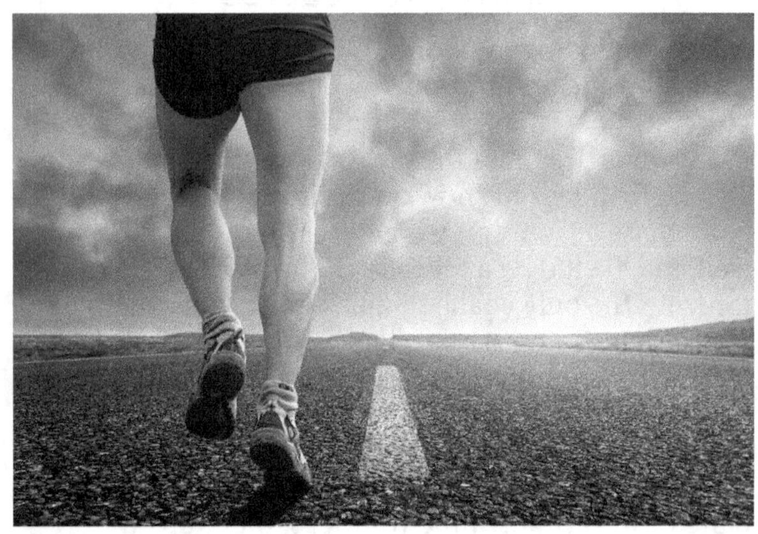

Straight Leg Lifts (Lying Down)

We'll use a mini-band for this exercise. If you have a physical therapy band, it may be possible to tie it in a loop that's an appropriate size to provide you with similar resistance to a mini-band.

Beginner: Use an 80 ounce (2,267 gram / 5 pound) resistance band. Or use a "light" weight band if yours don't have weights.

Advanced: Use a 160 ounce (4,535 gram / 10 pound) to a 320 ounce (9,071 gram / 20 pound) resistance band, or weights in that range. Or use "medium" to "heavy" weight bands.

Here's the process:

1. Place the mini-band around both legs just above your knees.
2. Lie down on your right side, supporting yourself on your right arm, which should be bent in an "L" so you can support your head with your hand. The rest of your body should be in a straight line.
3. Bend your right leg at a 90-degree angle so that your foot is pointing behind you. This will help with balance and form.
4. Make sure your hips stay square to the ground. Keep your left leg extended out straight and slowly lift it up to about a 45-degree angle.
5. Slowly lower your leg back down to the starting position.
6. Repeat this 15 to 20 times. Then, switch to your left side, and repeat the same with your right leg.

Side Steps (With Band Above Knee)

We'll use a mini-band again for this one! Or again, a physical therapy band if you can tie it securely in an appropriate loop.

Beginner: Use an 80 ounce (2,267 gram / 5 pound) resistance band. Or use a "light" weight band if yours don't have weights.

Advanced: Use a 160 ounce (4,535 gram / 10 pound) to a 320 ounce (9,071 gram / 20 pound) resistance band, or weights in that range. Or use "medium" to "heavy" weight bands.

Here's the process:

1. Start standing and circle your resistance band around both legs just above the knee. Scoot your feet shoulder-width apart, and keep your knees slightly bent.
2. Take a generous, slow, and controlled step to your right with your right leg, stretching the band as you go.
3. Now, follow with your left leg, coming back to a shoulder-width apart stance.
4. Next, take a generous step to your left with your left leg.
5. Follow with your right leg, coming back to your shoulder-width apart stance.
6. Repeat this 15 to 20 times.

Make sure when you're taking your steps that you keep the non-moving leg stable and square in the position it was when you started.

Additionally, make sure the leg you're moving stays nice and square with your bent knee facing straight out.

Don't let the resistance band pull your legs inward toward each other as you're trying to move! Try to keep a solid stance.

Side Steps (With Band Above Ankles)

Just like the last exercise, go with a mini-band or a physical therapy band tied in a loop.

Beginner: Use an 80 ounce (2,267 gram / 5 pound) resistance band. Or use a "light" weight band if yours don't have weights.

Advanced: Use a 160 ounce (4,535 gram / 10 pound) to a 320 ounce (9,071 gram / 20 pound) resistance band, or weights in that range. Or use "medium" to "heavy" weight bands.

Here's the process:

1. Start standing and circle your resistance band around both legs just above your ankles. Move your feet shoulder-width apart, keeping your knees slightly bent.
2. Take a generous step to your right with your right leg.
3. Follow along with your left leg until you're at your starting stance again.
4. Then, take a generous step to your left with your left leg.
5. Follow it with your right leg, returning to your starting stance.
6. Repeat this 15 to 20 times.

Standing Side Leg Lifts

Grab your mini-band or your physical therapy band tied in a loop.

Beginner: Use an 80 ounce (2,267 gram / 5 pound) resistance band. Or use a "light" weight band if yours don't have weights.

Advanced: Use a 160 ounce (4,535 gram / 10 pound) to a 320 ounce (9,071 gram / 20 pound) resistance band, or weights in that range. Or use "medium" to "heavy" weight bands.

Here's the process:

1. Circle your resistance band around both legs just above the ankles. Stand with your feet together.
2. Keeping your leg straight and knees just slightly bent (not locked), raise your right leg to your side, stretching the band as you go.
3. Slowly return to your starting position.
4. Repeat 15 to 20 times.
5. Switch to your left leg, and now repeat the same.

If balance is an issue, you can rest your hand lightly on a wall for support. Just make sure you're not leaning into your arm or using it to reduce the effectiveness of your exercise.

Single-Leg Extensions

Bonus! This one will also help work your abs. There are three different variations of this exercise.

The Mini-Band Supine Variation

Beginner: Use an 80 ounce (2,267 gram / 5 pound) resistance band. Or use a "light" weight band if yours don't have weights.

Advanced: Use a 160 ounce (4,535 gram / 10 pound) to a 320 ounce (9,071 gram / 20 pound) resistance band, or weights in that range. Or use "medium" to "heavy" weight bands.

1. Lie down on your back. Circle your band around both your feet, making sure to keep the band at the middle of your feet.
2. Bring both legs up to a 90-degree angle so that your thighs are vertical and your calves are parallel to the floor. (Keep those feet with the soles facing out away from you.)
3. Keep hip-distance between your legs so you can keep the band tight on your feet.
4. Extend your right leg out straight, at about a 45-degree angle, and keep your left leg in place as you do so (it's anchoring the band).
5. Hold for a few moments, then slowly return your right leg back to where it started.
6. Do the very same with the left leg extended now.
7. Repeat this 10 to 15 times.

The Alternate Supine Variation

You can use a power (loop) resistance band, tube resistance band, or physical therapy band for this version.

Beginner: Use a 48 ounce (1,360 gram / 3 pound) to an 80 ounce (2,267 gram / 5 pound) resistance band.

Advanced: Use a 160 ounce (4,535 gram / 10 pound) to a 320 ounce (9,071 gram / 20 pound) resistance band, or higher depending on your capability.

This version is also more friendly to those worried about their mini bands slipping off their feet.

1. Lie down on your back, with your legs bent (and your feet on the floor).
2. Loop your resistance band around the center of your right foot. To make sure you have enough resistance and to make sure your band is reliably anchored around your foot, you can wrap the band once around the foot completely first.
3. Bring your right leg up at a 90 degree angle so that your thigh is vertical and your calf is parallel with the floor.
4. Push your right leg out straight at a 45-degree angle.
5. Return your leg to the starting position. Repeat this 10 to 15 times.
6. Now, switch to your left leg, and do the same.

Seated Variation

Use a mini-band or a physical therapy band tied in a loop.

Beginner: Use an 80 ounce (2,267 gram / 5 pound) resistance band. Or use a "light" weight band if yours don't have weights.

Advanced: Use a 160 ounce (4,535 gram / 10 pound) to a 320 ounce (9,071 gram / 20 pound) resistance band, or weights in that range. Or use "medium" to "heavy" weight bands.

1. Start seated on the edge of a chair, with your legs just slightly apart.
2. Circle one end of the band above your right ankle and anchor the other end of the band around the right chair leg. Make sure you have a sturdy chair.
3. Extend your right leg out straight to a 45-degree angle.
4. Return to the starting position. Repeat this 10 to 15 times.
5. Now, switch to your left leg (and left chair leg with your band), and do the same.

Seated Hip Abduction

This exercise is best accomplished with a mini-band or a physical therapy band tied in a loop. However, it's also sometimes done with a tube resistance band wrapped around the legs a time or two to give the right resistance. It just might be less comfortable on your legs that way.

Beginner: Use an 80 ounce (2,267 gram / 5 pound) resistance band or lighter. Or use a "light" weight band if yours don't have weights.

Advanced: Use a 160 ounce (4,535 gram / 10 pound) to a 320 ounce (9,071 gram / 20 pound) resistance band, or weights in that range. Or use "medium" to "heavy" weight bands.

Here's the process:

1. Start seated on the edge of a chair, with your legs together.
2. Circle your resistance band around both legs just above the knee, or wrap your resistance band around both legs above the knee one or two times to get suitable resistance if you're using a tube resistance band.
3. Keeping your feet grounded together where they are and keeping your knees bent, pull your thighs apart from each other.
4. Make a controlled return to the starting position.
5. Repeat this 15 to 20 times.

Calves

Seated Toe Pushes

This exercise, along with many others intended to target the calves, does require you to loop the band around the balls of your feet, as opposed to the center where the band is most secure.

Normally this is something we'd caution against because it gives the band more opportunity to slip off. However, targeting the calves with resistance bands is most commonly done this way. So, for safety's sake, wear shoes (as always) and make sure you keep an eye on the band throughout the exercise to be aware of any slipping.

You can use these bands for this exercise:

- Power (loop) Resistance Band
- Physical Therapy Resistance Band
- Mini-Band

Beginner: Use a 48 ounce (1,360 gram / 3 pound) to an 80 ounce (2,267 gram / 5 pound) resistance band.

Advanced: Use a 160 ounce (4,535 gram / 10 pound) to a 320 ounce (9,071 gram / 20 pound) resistance band.

Here's the process:

1. Start seated on the floor, with your legs straight out in front of you. Keep your back straight.

2. Loop your resistance band around the balls of both feet, and hold the other end with both hands, drawing it taut enough to provide adequate resistance.
3. Tilt your foot forward from the ankle. You'll want to be sure you're flexing your calves while doing so.
4. Return to your starting position slowly.
5. Repeat this 15 to 25 times.

Calf Raise Side Steps With Resistance Band

Let's use a mini-band for this exercise. Fabric mini-bands can sometimes have a substantial width, so rubber mini-bands may work best here.

Beginner: Use an 80 ounce (2,267 gram / 5 pound) resistance band or lighter. Or use a "light" weight band if yours don't have weights.

Advanced: Use a 160 ounce (4,535 gram / 10 pound) to a 320 ounce (9,071 gram / 20 pound) resistance band, or weights in that range. Or use "medium" to "heavy" weight bands.

Here's the process:

1. Start standing, and loop your band around the middle of both feet.
2. Scoot out to a shoulder-width stance.
3. Raise yourself up on the balls of your feet, engaging your calves.

4. Take two steps to your right while on the balls of your feet. Make sure to keep your feet stable. Don't let the resistance band pull them in toward each other.
5. Now, take two steps back to your left.
6. Repeat 10 to 15 times.

If you're having trouble holding your balance, you can lightly rest your hands on a wall as you step.

Resistance Band Squatting Sole Raise

You can use a mini-band for this one or a physical therapy band tied in a loop. We won't lie; this exercise is definitely difficult, especially if you're also new to squatting. So, take it little by little!

Beginner: Use an 80 ounce (2,267 gram / 5 pound) resistance band or lighter. Or use a "light" weight band if yours don't have weights.

Advanced: Use a 160 ounce (4,535 gram / 10 pound) to a 320 ounce (9,071 gram / 20 pound) resistance band, or weights in that range. Or use "medium" to "heavy" weight bands.

Here's the process:

1. Start standing, and loop your band around both legs just above the knee.
2. Move your feet hip-width apart.

3. Come into a squatting position, and try to get your thighs as close to parallel with the ground as you can.
4. Now, come up onto the balls of both feet, and hold this for a moment or two.
5. Return your feet to the floor as slow and controlled as you can.
6. Repeat this 5 to 10 times, or more if your calves are up to it!

For this exercise, too, you can lightly rest your fingers on a wall to help with your balance.

Have your legs had enough yet? Well, they're not done! We're headed for those coveted glute-boosting exercises next, and often times exercises that engage your glutes also engage your thighs and even your calves. Your lower body tends to work best as a unit of combined strengths.

So, if you're looking for shapelier glutes, stronger glutes, lean muscular glutes, or all of the above, press on!

Chapter 8: Glute Strengthening Exercises

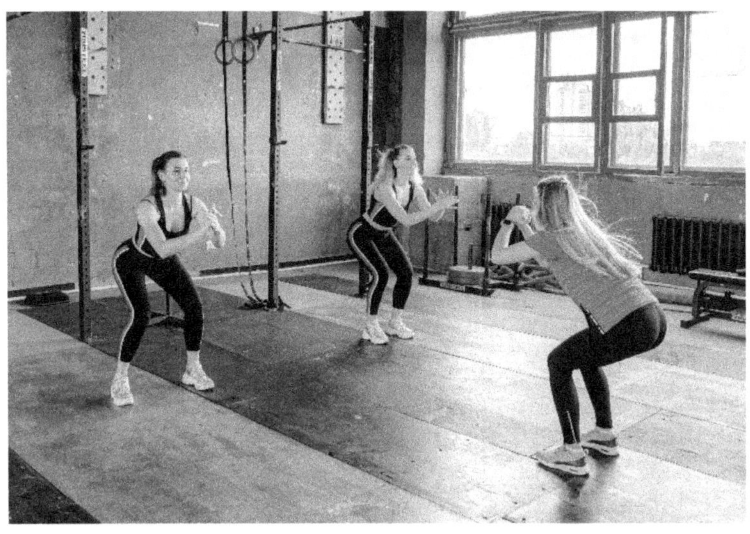

We're finally here. For those of us who are trying to get away from the dreaded "chair butt" that comes as a consequence of seated work, exercises that target and build the glutes are lifesavers.

Now, here's the answer to the big question. Can you get toned, muscular glutes without squats, squats, and more squats?

The easy answer is yes! We know that squats aren't for everyone, and they can be difficult if you suffer from knee pain. Thankfully, there are plenty of exercises that target the glutes. We're not going to stay away from squats altogether, but if you'd prefer to skip them for now, there are lots of other exercises available to get your glutes burning.

Now, mini-bands are called "booty bands" for a reason! Glute exercises are typically best done with a mini-band, so it's a worthy investment to have at least one on-hand.

Bridge Hold With Abduction

For this exercise, you can use:

- A mini-band.
- A physical therapy band tied in a loop.

Beginner: Use an 80 ounce (2,267 gram / 5 pound) resistance band or lighter. Or use a "light" weight band if yours don't have weights.

Advanced: Use a 160 ounce (4,535 gram / 10 pound) to a 320 ounce (9,071 gram / 20 pound) resistance band, or weights in that range. Or use "medium" to "heavy" weight bands.

Here's the process:

1. Lie down on your back on the floor, with your knees bent in front of you. Circle your resistance band around both legs just above the knee.
2. Scoot your legs hip-width apart.

3. Raise your bottom up until your body forms a straight descending line from your knees down to your shoulders.
4. Hold this position, and now pull your thighs apart slowly three times. You can roll your feet onto their sides to help this action, but try to keep your feet in the same place as they started. Don't take any steps.
5. Bring your bottom back down to your starting position.
6. Repeat this 10 to 15 times.

Standing Kickback

For this exercise, you can use:

- A mini-band.
- A physical therapy band tied in a loop.

Beginner: Use an 80 ounce (2,267 gram / 5 pound) resistance band or lighter. Or use a "light" weight band if yours don't have weights.

Advanced: Use a 160 ounce (4,535 gram / 10 pound) to a 320 ounce (9,071 gram / 20 pound) resistance band, or weights in that range. Or use "medium" to "heavy" weight bands.

Here's the process:

1. Start standing about hip-width apart, and loop your resistance band around both legs just above the ankles.

2. Move your right leg back a little and only have the ball of your foot touching the floor. Put all your weight on your left leg.
3. Move your right leg back about six inches, just so your foot leaves the floor.
4. Bring your right leg back in and return the ball of your foot to the floor.
5. Repeat 10 to 15 times.
6. Next, switch sides, and do the same with your left leg.

You can rest your hands on a nearby wall if needed for extra balance support.

Clamshells

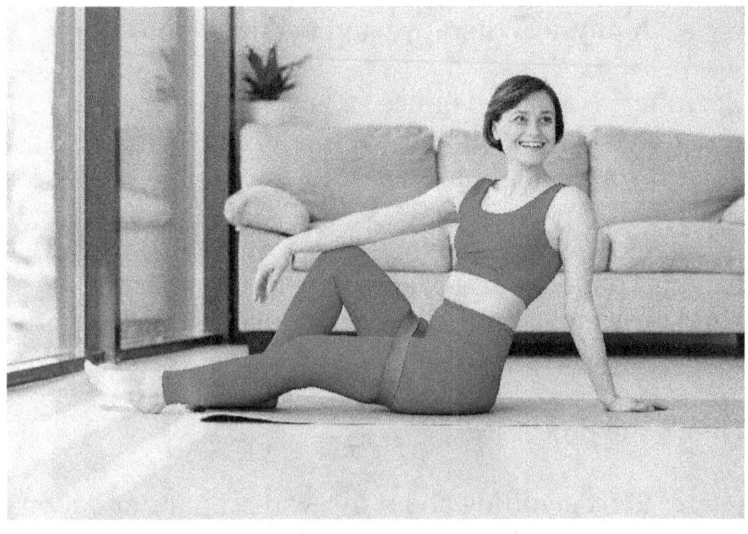

For this exercise, you can use:

- A mini-band.
- A physical therapy band tied in a loop.

Beginner: Use an 80 ounce (2,267 gram / 5 pound) resistance band or lighter. Or use a "light" weight band if yours don't have weights.

Advanced: Use a 160 ounce (4,535 gram / 10 pound) to a 320 ounce (9,071 gram / 20 pound) resistance band, or weights in that range. Or use "medium" to "heavy" weight bands.

Here's the process:

1. Lie down on the floor on your right side, with your knees bent and together, and hold your head up with your right arm.
2. Loop your resistance band around both legs
3. Bring both of your feet to about the height of your hip. Your right thigh should still be resting on the ground.
4. Keeping your feet together, pull your left knee away from your right knee.
5. Return your left knee slowly back down. Repeat 10 to 15 times.
6. Switch to your left side, and do the same with your left leg.

Hands and Knees Side Leg Raise

For this exercise, you can use:

- A mini-band.
- A physical therapy band tied in a loop.

Beginner: Use an 80 ounce (2,267 gram / 5 pound) resistance band or lighter. Or use a "light" weight band if yours don't have weights.

Advanced: Use a 160 ounce (4,535 gram / 10 pound) to a 320 ounce (9,071 gram / 20 pound) resistance band, or weights in that range. Or use "medium" to "heavy" weight bands.

Here's the process:

1. Start on the floor on your hands and knees, with your knees close together.
2. Loop your resistance band around both legs just above the knee.
3. Lift your right leg up to your side, aiming for about a 45-degree angle. Make sure to keep your hips straight and square as you do so.
4. Return your leg back down to its starting position. Repeat this 10 to 15 times.
5. Now, switch to your left leg and do the same.

Donkey Kicks

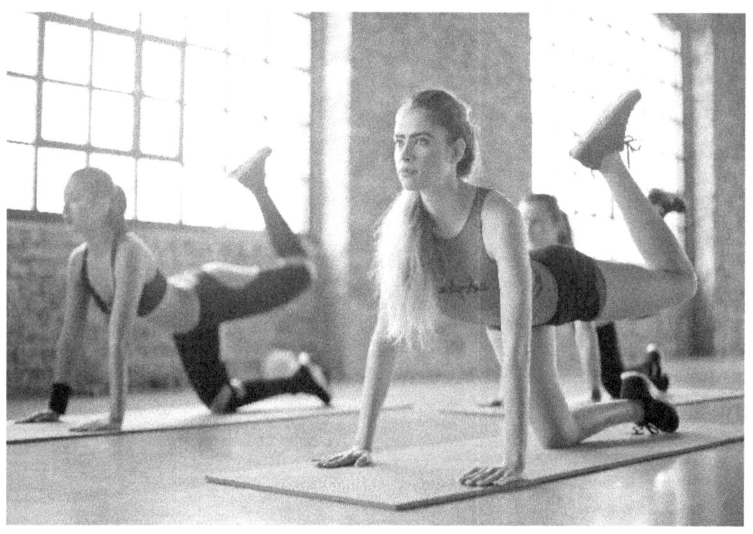

For this exercise, you can use:

- A mini-band.
- A physical therapy band tied in a loop.

Beginner: Use an 80 ounce (2,267 gram / 5 pound) resistance band or lighter. Or use a "light" weight band if yours don't have weights.

Advanced: Use a 160 ounce (4,535 gram / 10 pound) to a 320 ounce (9,071 gram / 20 pound) resistance band, or weights in that range. Or use "medium" to "heavy" weight bands.

Here's the process:

1. Start on your hands and knees, with your knees about hip-width apart.
2. Loop your resistance band around both legs just above the knee.
3. Lift your right leg up behind you so that your thigh is parallel to the floor. Your knee should stay bent, so the soles of your feet should be facing the ceiling.
4. Hold for a moment at the top, then bring your leg slowly back down.
5. Now, switch to your right leg and do the same.
6. Repeat 10 to 15 times.

Supine Clamshell

For this exercise, you can use:

- A mini-band.
- A physical therapy band tied in a loop.

Beginner: Use an 80 ounce (2,267 gram / 5 pound) resistance band or lighter. Or use a "light" weight band if yours don't have weights.

Advanced: Use a 160 ounce (4,535 gram / 10 pound) to a 320 ounce (9,071 gram / 20 pound) resistance band, or weights in that range. Or use "medium" to "heavy" weight bands.

Here's the process:

1. Lie down on your back, and loop your band around both legs just above the knee.
2. Bend both legs so that your thighs are vertical and your calves are parallel with the floor.
3. Pull your knees in just a little further toward your chest. You don't want to be hugging them; you just want to make sure your knees are a bit above your hip line.
4. Start with your knees together. Then, pull your thighs apart from each other until your knees are just about shoulder-width apart.
5. Return to the starting position slowly, with your knees together.
6. Repeat this 10 to 15 times.

Banded Squats

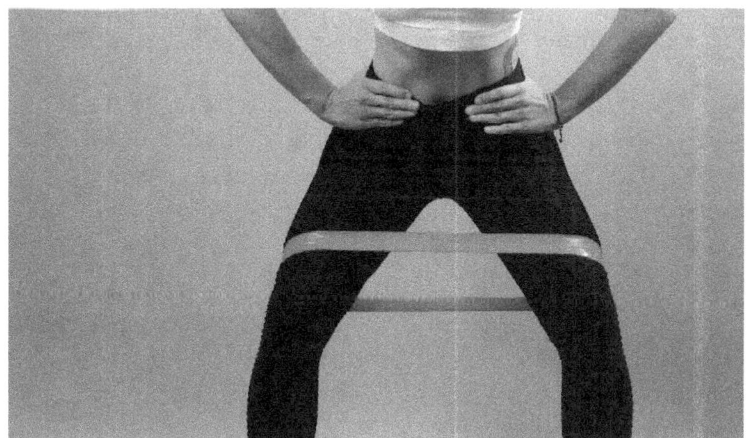

For this exercise, you can use:

- A mini-band.
- A physical therapy band tied in a loop.

Beginner: Use an 80 ounce (2,267 gram / 5 pound) resistance band or lighter. Or use a "light" weight band if yours don't have weights.

Advanced: Use a 160 ounce (4,535 gram / 10 pound) to a 320 ounce (9,071 gram / 20 pound) resistance band, or weights in that range. Or use "medium" to "heavy" weight bands.

Here's the process:

1. Start standing, and loop your band around both legs just above the knees.
2. Move your feet out to shoulder width, with your toes facing just slightly outward.
3. Squat down until your thighs are about parallel with the floor. It's okay if your torso is slanted slightly forward; just make sure that you're keeping the line of your back nice and straight.
4. Hold the squat for a moment, then return to the starting stand.
5. Repeat 10 to 15 times.

To help with balance, squats are often done with arms extended straight out in front of you while in the squatting position. If you need to touch a wall for balance support, do so!

Monster Walks

For this exercise, you can use:

- A mini-band.
- A physical therapy band tied in a loop.

Beginner: Use an 80 ounce (2,267 gram / 5 pound) resistance band or lighter. Or use a "light" weight band if yours don't have weights.

Advanced: Use a 160 ounce (4,535 gram / 10 pound) to a 320 ounce (9,071 gram / 20 pound) resistance band, or weights in that range. Or use "medium" to "heavy" weight bands.

Here's the process:

1. Start standing, and loop your band around both legs just above the ankles.
2. Move your feet shoulder-width apart, with your toes just slightly turned outward.
3. Come to a partial squat. Your thighs don't need to be parallel with the floor, just about halfway there.
4. Hold your hands together in front of you and walk forward, slowly and stable.
5. Aim to walk from one end of the room to the other and return again. If you're not feeling the burn yet, or if you have a short room, do another 1 to 2 rounds.

Side Lunge With Kick

For this exercise, you can use:

- A mini-band.
- A physical therapy band tied in a loop.

Beginner: Use an 80 ounce (2,267 gram / 5 pound) resistance band or lighter. Or use a "light" weight band if yours don't have weights.

Advanced: Use a 160 ounce (4,535 gram / 10 pound) to a 320 ounce (9,071 gram / 20 pound) resistance band, or weights in that range. Or use "medium" to "heavy" weight bands.

Here's the process:

1. Start standing and loop your band around both legs just above the knee.
2. Scoot your feet shoulder-width apart.
3. Move your right leg further out to the side and bend it at the knee until your thigh is about halfway to parallel with the floor. Keep your left leg straight and in place as you lunge.
4. Return to the starting position.
5. Still, with your right leg, lift it up at your side to about a 45-degree angle, then return to the starting position again.
6. Repeat this 10 to 15 times, lunging, then kicking, lunging, then kicking.
7. Next, do the same, lunge and kick with your left leg 10 to 15 times.

Bridge Pulses

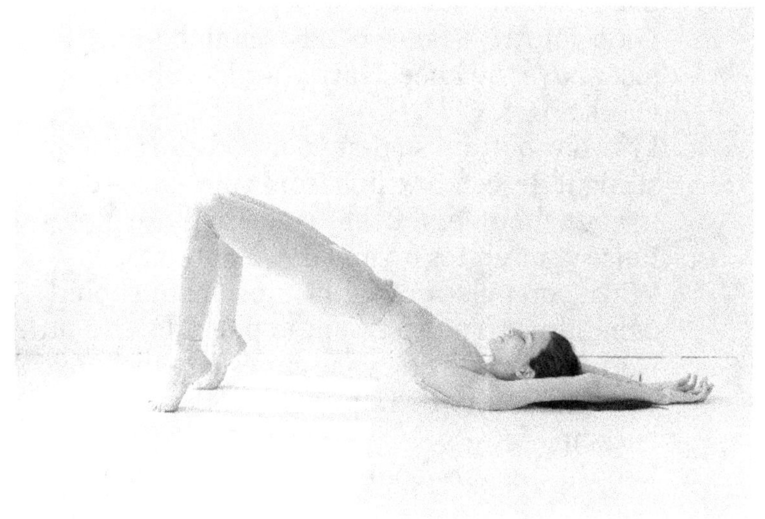

For this exercise, you can use:

- A mini-band.
- A physical therapy band tied in a loop.

Beginner: Use an 80 ounce (2,267 gram / 5 pound) resistance band or lighter. Or use a "light" weight band if yours don't have weights.

Advanced: Use a 160 ounce (4,535 gram / 10 pound) to a 320 ounce (9,071 gram / 20 pound) resistance band, or weights in that range. Or use "medium" to "heavy" weight bands.

Here's the process:

1. Lie down on your back with your knees bent. Loop your resistance band around both legs just above the knee. Have your feet about hip-width apart.
2. Lift your bottom so that your body forms a straight descending line from your knees down to your shoulders. Really squeeze those glutes.
3. Pulse your glutes up and down at the top. When you pulse down, the movement should be minimal. You just want to pulse down a little while still squeezing your glutes and then give your glutes an extra squeeze when you pulse back up.
4. Keep at this for about 30 seconds to 1 minute.

If your buns are burning just reading this, then good!

Chapter 9: Recovery

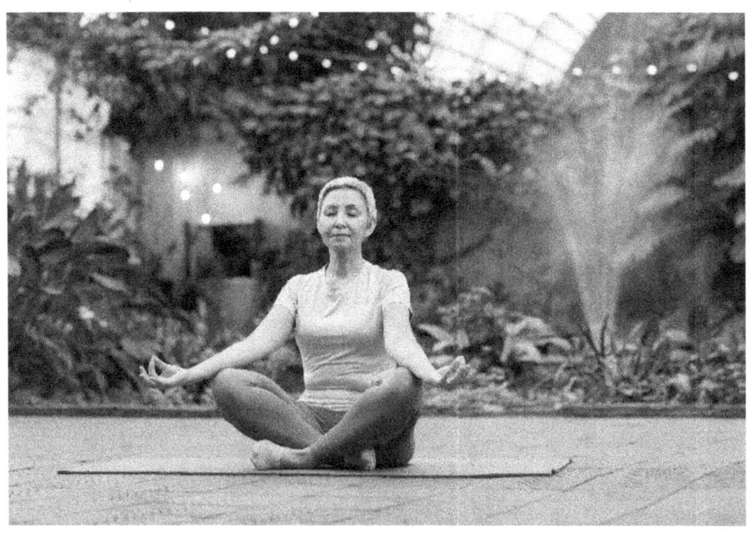

As much as any of us might just wish we could grit our teeth, go gung-ho every day of the week and get this path to a stronger body "over with," taking time to rest and recover is non-negotiable.

Our bodies don't respond well to repeated, intense physical stress on the same muscle groups day after day, and the reason for this is the way our bodies repair themselves after exercise.

During your exercises, your muscle fibers are consistently tearing on a microscopic level. Don't be alarmed! This is what leads to post-exercise muscle soreness and is completely normal. The microscopic tears that your muscles endure are what lead to stronger muscles in the future.

It's during your recovery time after exercise when you're binge-watching shows, sleeping, and becoming one with your couch that your muscles are becoming bigger and better. After your muscles have torn, they can take 24 to 48 hours to knit back together stronger than they were before.

The recovery phase is essential to this process. If you're constantly working the same muscle groups day after day, your muscles will tear and then tear again and tear again, leading to continual breakdown without enough time to repair. This doesn't build those stronger muscles that you're looking for and isn't conducive to a healthier body or lifestyle.

We know what you're thinking. How can I establish a consistent routine if I'm working one day and lazing out the next? The answer to that is simple. Cycle your exercise circuits! Resting your muscles doesn't mean you have to be inactive. Work out one group of muscles one day, and the next day, work a different group of muscles while your first muscle group rests.

Or, it's perfectly fine to have one day on, one day off from your intense muscle-building exercises. You can still develop a strong routine this way. Plus, your off-days don't mean you have to laze around doing no activity at all. To keep up with your routine of daily activity, you can do some light, soothing activity, like walking or yoga, on your days "off."

Now, here are some essential tips to helping your muscles recover faster, whether you're on an off-day or whether you're cycling through to other muscle groups. Most of them are easy habits to adopt and take hardly any time at all.

Eat Your High Protein Foods Soon After Exercise

It's been proven that eating soon after exercise can actually be extremely beneficial for your muscles, but you do have to eat the right things.

We know for some, this may be off-putting. Eating before exercise and then exercising hoping to burn off the calories you just took in isn't the best strategy and will often just leave you hungry sooner, making it more difficult for you to get to your next meal without giving in to snack temptations. Plus, it doesn't provide your muscles with the important after-workout nutrients they need to help them repair.

Generally, it's recommended to eat high-protein foods after exercise, and this has the best effect when you eat within an hour after working out. Think eggs, milk, yogurt, nuts, beans, and lean meats.

You'll also want to include some healthy carbohydrates into your after-workout meal. While protein helps your muscles repair themselves, carbohydrates help restore your energy reserves. Go for foods like an apple, a banana, oats, rice, or granola.

Catch Some Z's

This is probably one of the simplest ways you can help your body recover. We know everyone sleeps, but what we mean is to make sure you're getting *enough* sleep. That's 6 hours at least, up to the full 8 hours at night. An hour to an hour and a half afternoon nap can also be sprinkled in if you have the opportunity.

Have a fairly regular bedtime, don't stay up late into the wee hours of the morning if you can avoid it, and put those blue-light emitting phones away at least an hour before bed to ensure you're getting good, restful sleep. Good sleep isn't just about the hours, it's about the quality, and if you're having a fitful rest thanks to late social media wandering, you're not doing your body any favors.

Drink Your Water

How many times have you heard this one throughout your life? The truth is, most people don't drink enough water. Staying well-hydrated is another really good way to help your body to a speedy recovery.

Men need around 3.7 liters of water on average in a day. Women need around 2.7 liters.

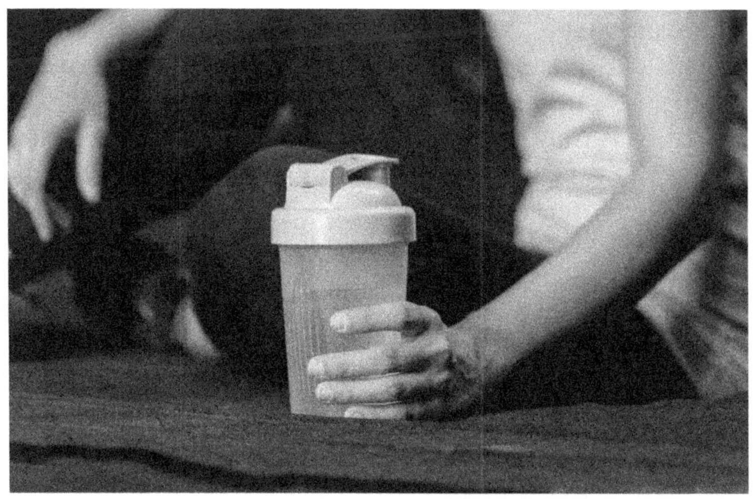

If you have trouble keeping track, there are plenty of water bottles and jugs on the market with measurement marks on the side to help you get your full intake.

Fight Soreness

Muscle soreness is the worst! Sometimes, there's just nothing much you can do about it if it's really intense. There are, however, some tried and true methods that can help ease this soreness at the moment and may even help it go away faster for some.

Stretch

Stretching is a very important tool to use both immediately after exercise and when muscle soreness is bothering you the day after.

Find easy stretches that target the muscles you just worked, and use them as your cool-down. This can help loosen up and get the blood flowing to those muscles. It may not always get rid of soreness, but it can at the very least lessen it and sometimes actually does prevent it altogether.

When you're already sore, choose some nice gentle stretches for your sore muscles and really invest the time into them. Do deep breathing as you stretch.

Use Moist Heat

Whenever there's pain in any form, it's really tempting to go straight to ice. Ice, however, is a better tool for injury recovery. For standard muscle soreness, moist heat can be a really effective tool for loosening and relaxing muscles and increasing blood flow to the area. The moistness element of the heat helps it penetrate deep into your muscles, where you need it most.

Moist heat is a great tool to use both immediately after exercise and during delayed onset soreness. Look for heat pads that can be converted to moist heat by spraying water on the surface. There are also moist heat pads that draw moisture from the air to produce moist heat and some that you can microwave, which produce moist heat.

Massage the Area

Right after you exercise, if you're able to massage the muscles you worked, then do! First of all, it'll feel amazing. Who doesn't long for a nice massage?

If you don't have the magic masseuse capabilities of a friend or partner to reach difficult-to-massage areas, you can buy a foam roller or a plastic muscle roller to help you get a good muscle massage. A tennis ball is another great tool to use to roll around under your muscles for a nice massage, and it's something more of us are more likely to already have. Your dog might not like it, but hey, they can share.

Acknowledge Injury, and Take Time to Heal

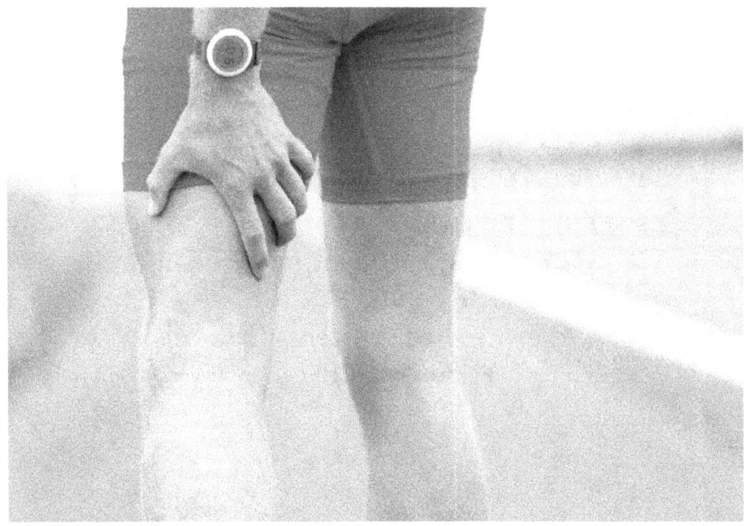

Muscle soreness may seem like an injury, but in truth, it's really not. Your muscle fibers have torn and are repairing, and this is a normal process that your body should take care of within 48 hours.

However, an injury has occurred when you are experiencing pain that is unlike muscle soreness. This can be a sharp or stabbing pain, a pulling pain, a dull ache, joint pain, etcetera. If what you thought was muscle soreness is severe persists too long to be normal, this may be a sign of injury as well.

Some injuries can be treated at home with time and care. Here are some things you can try to help yourself recover.

RICE

This may sound familiar. ICE is an acronym, which stands for the following:

- "R" – Rest. Relax, get your sleep, and don't work the injured area.
- "I" – Ice the injured area. This helps reduce swelling and ease the pain.
- "C" – Compression. Compress the injured area with an elastic bandage.
- "E" – Elevate the limb. This helps circulate blood and reduce swelling.

Epsom Salt Baths

Also a good solution for regular muscle soreness, Epsom salts can help reduce pain from minor injuries.

It's good to note that the benefits of Epsom salts haven't been proven per se, but Epsom salt baths have been a popular household remedy for a long time. Apart from the warm bath water, which will also help ease muscle and joint pains, Epsom salts dissolve into sulfate and magnesium in the water. It's thought that the magnesium can be absorbed via your skin and that this has something to do with pain relief.

Epsom salts are easy to find at most drugstores.

If All Else Fails...

See your doctor. If you don't seem to be getting any better after a week or two, something more serious may be going on, so a doctor's visit is in order.

Chapter 10: Weekly Workout Plans and Goal Setting

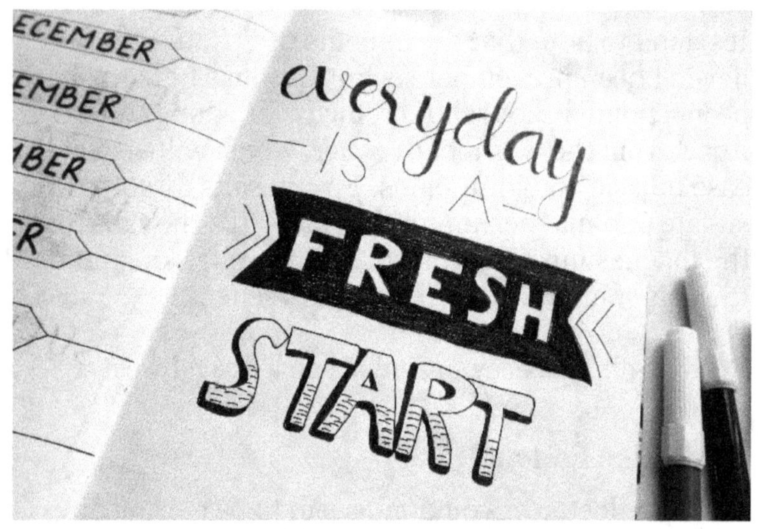

Being able to customize your own workout plan to your own needs can be a very rewarding and beneficial process, and we encourage it! But for many of us, trying to decide where to start can be a little daunting. So, we've put together some basic weekly workouts to give you somewhere to start and help you build a foundation for your own customized workout plans.

We've set out both a beginner and an advanced weekly workout plan, but we acknowledge that everyone's starting point is on a different level. Our version of beginner is light, but if it's not light enough, we encourage you to cut back on your repetitions or number of exercises until you're stronger. If it's too light and advanced is too heavy, strive for a customized number of reps in between the two.

Beginner – Week 1 and 2

For beginners, we want to try starting you off on a 3 day per week muscle training exercise schedule and go up from there, but we will provide optional day plans for the 4th, 5th, and 6th days. Again, training 3 days per week doesn't mean you have to be inactive on the "off" days. You can always toggle to a walk, yoga, or a light bike ride on your off days to keep up with your routine. We do, however, recommend you have at least one day of only rest per week.

We're cycling muscle groups, too, for full-body benefit while giving the muscle groups you've worked time to rest the next day. So, how you pace out these days in your week is up to you. You can do them in tandem, one day after the other. Or, you can space them out with one day of light or no activity in between, depending on what you need.

Use lightweight bands for weeks 1 and 2.

Day 1 – Arms and Shoulders

Bicep Curl – 5 reps, each arm.
Shrug – 10 reps.
Pull-Apart – 10 reps.
Behind Pull-Apart – 10 reps.
Overhead Press – 10 reps.

Upright Row – 5 reps.
Bent Lift – 5 reps.

Day 2 – Abs, Back, and Chest

Standing twist – 10 reps.
Supine Chest Press – 10 reps.
Deadlift – 5 reps.
Resistance Band Russian Twist – 10 reps.
Standing Incline Press – 10 reps.
Plank Kick – 5 reps, each leg.
Resistance Band Push Ups – 3 reps.
Bent Back Fly – 10 reps.

Day 3 – Legs and Glutes

Side Steps (band above the knee) – 10 reps.
Single-Leg Extensions – 10 reps, each leg.
Clamshell – 10 reps, each leg.
Banded Squats – 5 reps.
Standing Side Leg Lifts – 5 reps, each leg.
Monster Walks – 1 full trip across the room and back.
Bridge Hold with Abduction – 5 reps.
Resistance Band Squatting Sole Raise – 3 reps.

Day 4 (optional) – Arms and Shoulders

Bicep Curl – 5 reps, each arm.
Shrug – 10 reps.
Pull-Apart – 10 reps.
Behind Pull Apart – 10 reps.
Overhead Press – 10 reps.
Upright Row – 5 reps.
Bent Lift – 5 reps.

Day 5 (optional) – Abs, Back, and Chest

Standing twist – 10 reps.
Supine Chest Press – 10 reps.
Deadlift – 5 reps.
Resistance Band Russian Twist – 10 reps.
Standing Incline Press – 10 reps.
Plank Kick – 5 reps, each leg.
Resistance Band Push Ups – 3 reps.
Bent Back Fly – 10 reps.

Day 6 (optional) – Legs and Glutes

Side Steps (band above the knee) – 10 reps.
Single-Leg Extensions – 10 reps, each leg.
Clamshell – 10 reps, each leg.
Banded Squats – 5 reps.
Standing Side Leg Lifts – 5 reps, each leg.
Monster Walks – 1 full trip across the room and back.
Bridge Hold with Abduction – 5 reps.
Resistance Band Squatting Sole Raise – 3 reps.

Beginner – Week 3 and 4

Stay on a lightweight band if you need to, or move up one step to a heavier band if you're up for the challenge.

Day 1 – Arms and Shoulders

Bicep Curl – 8 reps, each arm.
Shrug – 15 reps.

Pull-Apart – 12 reps.
Behind Pull Apart – 12 reps.
Overhead Press – 12 reps.
Upright Row – 8 reps.
Bent Lift – 8 reps.
Front Raise – 5 reps.

Day 2 – Abs, Back, and Chest

Standing twist – 12 reps.
Supine Chest Press – 12 reps.
Deadlift – 8 reps.
Resistance Band Russian Twist – 12 reps.
Standing Incline Press – 12 reps.
Plank Kick – 8 reps, each leg.
Resistance Band Push Ups – 5 reps.
Bent Back Fly – 12 reps.
Seated Resistance Band Rows – 10 reps.

Day 3 – Legs and Glutes

Side Steps (band above the ankle) – 15 reps.
Single-Leg Extensions – 15 reps, each leg.
Supine Clamshell – 12 reps, each leg.
Banded Squats – 8 reps.
Donkey Kicks – 8 reps, each leg.
Monster Walks – 2 full trips across the room and back.
Bridge Hold with Abduction – 8 reps.
Bridge Pulses – 5 reps.
Resistance Band Squatting Sole Raise – 5 reps.

Day 4 (optional) – Arms and Shoulders

Bicep Curl – 8 reps, each arm.
Shrug – 15 reps.
Pull-Apart – 12 reps.
Behind Pull Apart – 12 reps.
Overhead Press – 12 reps.
Upright Row – 8 reps.
Bent Lift – 8 reps.
Front Raise – 5 reps.

Day 5 (optional) – Abs, Back, and Chest

Standing twist – 12 reps.
Supine Chest Press – 12 reps.
Deadlift – 8 reps.
Resistance Band Russian Twist – 12 reps.
Standing Incline Press – 12 reps.
Plank Kick – 8 reps, each leg.
Resistance Band Push Ups – 5 reps.
Bent Back Fly – 12 reps.
Seated Resistance Band Rows – 10 reps.

Day 6 (optional) – Legs and Glutes

Side Steps (band above the ankle) – 15 reps.
Single-Leg Extensions – 15 reps, each leg.
Supine Clamshell – 12 reps, each leg.
Banded Squats – 8 reps.
Donkey Kicks – 8 reps, each leg.
Monster Walks – 2 full trips across the room and back.
Bridge Hold with Abduction – 8 reps.
Bridge Pulses – 5 reps.

Resistance Band Squatting Sole Raise – 5 reps.

Advanced – Week 1 and 2

Now, we're cranking up the challenge a lot here to provide a workout that gives enough difficulty for those who are already used to exercise or who have already strengthened their muscles quite a bit.

Jumping from beginner to advanced might be a bit of a shock, so be sure to assess your abilities and take it slow when deciding to move from beginner to advanced. You can always adjust the reps and the weight of your band to fall somewhere in between, giving you a more relaxed bridge up to the advanced plan.

Use medium-weight bands for weeks 1 and two.

Day 1 – Arms and Shoulders

Bicep Curl – 15 reps, each arm.
Shrug – 20 reps.
Pull-Apart – 20 reps.
Behind Pull Apart – 20 reps.
Overhead Press – 20 reps.
Upright Row – 15 reps.
Bent Lift – 15 reps.

Day 2 – Abs, Back, and Chest

Standing twist – 20 reps.
Supine Chest Press – 20 reps.

Deadlift – 15 reps.
Resistance Band Russian Twist – 20 reps.
Standing Incline Press – 20 reps.
Plank Kick – 15 reps, each leg.
Resistance Band Push Ups – 15 reps.
Bent Back Fly – 20 reps.

Day 3 – Legs and Glutes

Side Steps (band above the knee) – 20 reps.
Single-Leg Extensions – 20 reps, each leg.
Clamshell – 20 reps, each leg.
Banded Squats – 15 reps.
Standing Side Leg Lifts – 15 reps, each leg.
Monster Walks – 4 full trips across the room and back.
Bridge Hold with Abduction – 15 reps.
Resistance Band Squatting Sole Raise – 10 reps.
Calf Raise Side Steps – 10 reps.

Day 4 (optional) – Arms and Shoulders

Bicep Curl – 15 reps, each arm.
Shrug – 20 reps.
Pull-Apart – 20 reps.
Behind Pull Apart – 20 reps.
Overhead Press – 20 reps.
Upright Row – 15 reps.
Bent Lift – 15 reps.

Day 5 (optional) – Abs, Back, and Chest

Standing twist – 20 reps.
Supine Chest Press – 20 reps.

Deadlift – 15 reps.
Resistance Band Russian Twist – 20 reps.
Standing Incline Press – 20 reps.
Plank Kick – 15 reps, each leg.
Resistance Band Push Ups – 15 reps.
Bent Back Fly – 20 reps.

Day 6 (optional) – Legs and Glutes

Side Steps (band above the knee) – 20 reps.
Single-Leg Extensions – 20 reps, each leg.
Clamshell – 20 reps, each leg.
Banded Squats – 15 reps.
Standing Side Leg Lifts – 15 reps, each leg.
Monster Walks – 4 full trips across the room and back.
Bridge Hold with Abduction – 15 reps.
Resistance Band Squatting Sole Raise – 10 reps.
Calf Raise Side Steps – 10 reps.

Advanced – Week 3 and 4

Now, you can stay on your medium-weight band if it's still giving you enough challenge, or you can move up to a heavier weight band.

Day 1 – Arms and Shoulders

Bicep Curl – 20 reps, each arm.
Shrug – 25 reps.
Pull-Apart – 25 reps.
Behind Pull Apart – 25 reps.
Overhead Press – 25 reps.

Upright Row – 20 reps.
Bent Lift – 20 reps.

Day 2 – Abs, Back, and Chest

Standing twist – 25 reps.
Supine Chest Press – 25 reps.
Deadlift – 20 reps.
Resistance Band Russian Twist – 25 reps.
Standing Incline Press – 25 reps.
Plank Kick – 20 reps, each leg.
Resistance Band Push Ups – 20 reps.
Bent Back Fly – 25 reps.

Day 3 – Legs and Glutes

Side Steps (band above the knee) – 25 reps.
Single-Leg Extensions – 25 reps, each leg.
Clamshell – 25 reps, each leg.
Banded Squats – 20 reps.
Standing Side Leg Lifts – 20 reps, each leg.
Monster Walks – 6 full trips across the room and back.
Bridge Hold with Abduction – 20 reps.
Resistance Band Squatting Sole Raise – 15 reps.
Calf Raise Side Steps – 15 reps.

Day 4 (optional) – Arms and Shoulders

Bicep Curl – 20 reps, each arm.
Shrug – 25 reps.
Pull-Apart – 25 reps.
Behind Pull Apart – 25 reps.
Overhead Press – 25 reps.

Upright Row – 20 reps.
Bent Lift – 20 reps.

Day 5 (optional) – Abs, Back, and Chest

Standing twist – 25 reps.
Supine Chest Press – 25 reps.
Deadlift – 20 reps.
Resistance Band Russian Twist – 25 reps.
Standing Incline Press – 25 reps.
Plank Kick – 25 reps, each leg.
Resistance Band Push Ups – 20 reps.
Bent Back Fly – 25 reps.

Day 6 (optional) – Legs and Glutes

Side Steps (band above the knee) – 25 reps.
Single-Leg Extensions – 25 reps, each leg.
Clamshell – 25 reps, each leg.
Banded Squats – 20 reps.
Standing Side Leg Lifts – 20 reps, each leg.
Monster Walks – 6 full trips across the room and back.
Bridge Hold with Abduction – 20 reps.
Resistance Band Squatting Sole Raise – 15 reps.
Calf Raise Side Steps – 13 reps.

Bonus Plans For the Booty Only

Above, we've designed more of a full-body approach to our workout plans, but we know that for some, it's more of a priority to work one muscle group consistently. It's a personal choice what parts of the body you want to work and don't want to work, and we totally get that.

Many of you might be here looking for the booty shaping and boosting effects of resistance bands more than the full-body effect, so here, we've included some weekly plans that focus only on those glute blasting exercises.

Beginner – Week 1 and 2

Start with a lightweight band for week 1. For week 2, either stay with the lightweight band or move up to a medium weight.

Aim to accomplish this circuit at least 3 days per week, but make sure you give yourself at least 1 day of break in between to allow your muscles to heal. On your days off, do some yoga or go for a walk. Allow yourself one day of total rest each week.

Standing Kick Back – 10 reps, each leg.
Clamshell – 10 reps, each side.
Banded Squats – 5 reps.
Hands and Knees Side Leg Raise – 10 reps, each leg.
Bridge Pulses – 10 pulses.
Donkey Kicks – 10 reps, each leg.

Beginner – Week 2 and 3

Try to move up to a medium-weight band for weeks 2 and 3. Of course, if you feel that you should still stay on the lightweight band, do so!

Standing Kick Back – 15 reps, each leg.
Clamshell – 15 reps, each side.
Banded Squats – 8 reps.
Hands and Knees Side Leg Raise – 15 reps, each leg.
Bridge Pulses – 15 pulses.
Donkey Kicks – 15 reps, each leg.
Monster Walks – 1 trip across the room and back.
Bridge Hold with Abduction – 5 reps.

Advanced – Week 1 and 2

Start off with a medium-weight band for weeks 1 and 2.

Standing Kick Back – 20 reps, each leg.
Clamshell – 20 reps, each side.
Banded Squats – 12 reps.
Hands and Knees Side Leg Raise – 20 reps, each leg.
Bridge Pulses – 20 pulses.
Donkey Kicks – 20 reps, each leg.
Monster Walks – 3 trips across the room and back.
Bridge Hold with Abduction – 20 reps.
Side Lunge with Kick – 20 reps, each leg.
Supine Clamshell – 15 reps.

Advanced – Week 3 and 4

Go up to a heavyweight band for weeks 3 and 4.

Standing Kick Back – 25 reps, each leg.
Clamshell – 25 reps, each side.
Banded Squats – 15 reps.

Hands and Knees Side Leg Raise – 25 reps, each leg.
Bridge Pulses – 25 pulses.
Donkey Kicks – 25 reps, each leg.
Monster Walks – 5 trips across the room and back.
Bridge Hold with Abduction – 25 reps.
Side Lunge with Kick – 25 reps, each leg.
Supine Clamshell – 20 reps.

Goal Setting

When it comes to setting goals for yourself, there's really no one universal template to follow. Your goals must deeply reflect you and your understanding of yourself, not necessarily someone else's understanding of you.

There are, however, some important goal-setting tips you can follow that will help you make the wisest and most beneficial goals for your body.

Set Realistic, Achievable Goals

Trying to blast every pocket of fat from your entire body in 30 days or less, for instance, is not a realistic goal and not one that is achievable. Trying to make it so you can fit into a wedding dress two sizes too small in two weeks wouldn't be, either.

There are so many videos out there that encourage jumping into an exercise routine that's too difficult for beginners and pushing the 30-day "belly blast" or the "booty blast." While it seems like these types of exercise plans make short-term goals feel more achievable, they are often easy to drop because they start at a difficulty level far from suited for everyone. They also insist on a "push through and get it over with" type mentality, which doesn't foster an activity plan that lasts.

Set goals for yourself that start at a level you're comfortable with and that gradually increase the challenge at a reasonable pace for your body, allowing yourself recovery and rest days.

Be in It for the Long Run

It's perfectly fine to set some short-term goals along the way, don't get us wrong. These short-term goals, however, need to work up to a long-term goal, and when that long-term goal is met, a new long-term goal should already be set.

Make exercising regularly and improving your strength a lifestyle, not a fad. For an active routine to stick and to prevent the "slingshot" effect that occurs after short-term diet or exercise blasts are over, the exercise goals you set for yourself need to be a consistent part of your life.

Make Your Goals Specific

Don't be too vague when identifying what you want from your exercise. Be clear about what you want in terms of numbers and deadlines. For example, saying "I want to lose weight" is a good start, but we need to be more specific than that.

Keeping it realistic, a more specific version of this goal would be "I want to lose 4 pounds in the month of February."

Here, you've established a weight loss goal in terms of numbers and a deadline by which you'd like to achieve it, and this is the definition of a solid, realistic, and specific goal.

Personalize Your Goals

Following trends never does anyone any favors. Watching the acclaim and results of other people doing a workout plan online and what their goals were brings unhealthy comparisons into the picture. It forces us to strive for what worked for someone else and often causes us to fall prey to a negative body image and bitterness if we can't achieve the exact same results in the exact same amount of time.

So set goals that are yours, not someone else's. Base your goals on your body, your strength, and your capability. Work on meeting your own customized standards for yourself, and you're bound to have a much more positive outlook on your progress.

Don't Center Your Goals Around Negativity

You never want to approach new exercise goals with the mindset of "I hate my body, and I want it to change." Exercising out of hatred for an aspect of your body encourages a vicious cycle of negativity, leading to a warped view of ourselves. This makes exercise something we do out of anger or self-resentment, which defeats the "healthier life" that it's intended to help you achieve.

Set goals around positive thoughts, like, "I love my body, and I want to nourish it." "I want to push it to be stronger." "I want to put in the work to help it achieve more." Make your exercise goals an investment in self-love.

Don't Depend on the Scale

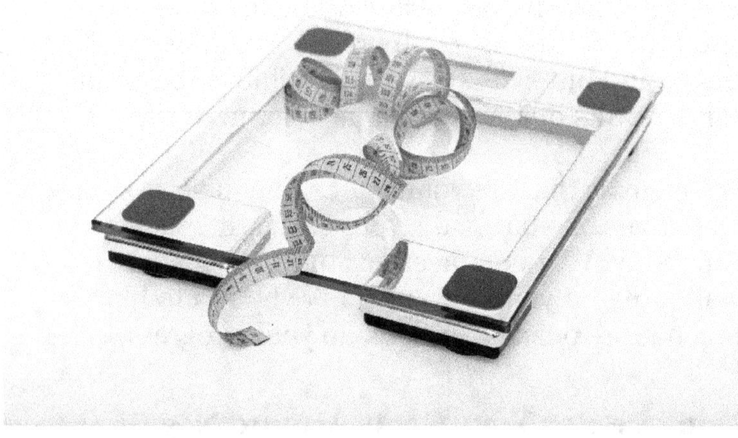

Contrary to popular belief, no, your bathroom scale doesn't determine how your exercise routine is working or whether you've met your goals or missed them. Some people even believe that we shouldn't own scales, because it tends to encourage an unhealthy addiction to the number as a definition of our self-worth.

It's certainly fine to have weight loss goals, but it's best to approach these goals from a point of view that extends past the scale. Your weight is made up of many complex factors. When we're talking about losing weight, we're talking about shedding fat mass in our body, but the scale's not just telling you how much your fat weighs.

If you're working on building muscle, always know that muscle weighs more than fat. So if you've made some serious muscle gains from your exercise goals, you may even see the number on the scale go up after a while rather than down.

To get a better overall idea of your progress, measure your waist, take notice of differences in how your clothes fit, note differences in the appearance of your lean muscle and silhouette. Most importantly, take stock of how you feel. How much effort you put into sticking to your goals is worth more than the number on the scale.

Chapter 11: Eating Your Way to a Healthier Lifestyle

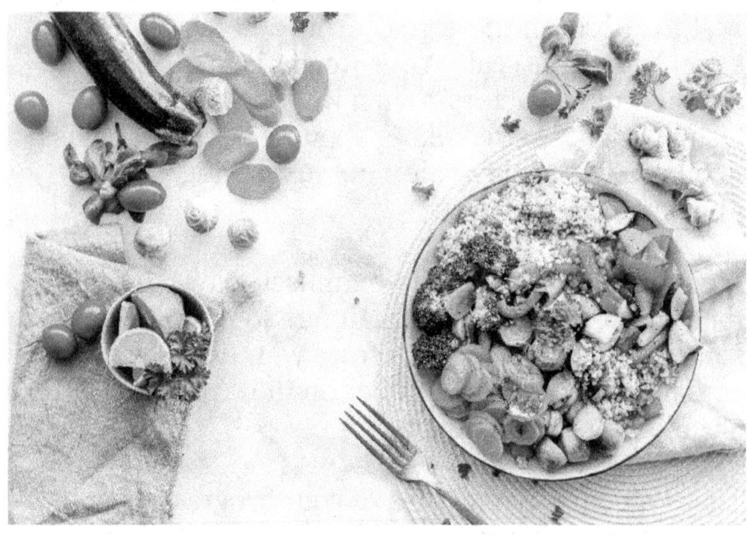

Starting an active routine is definitely a big breakthrough in changing your life for the better! It really is only half the battle, though.

We're sorry to say that exercising regularly doesn't open the doors to allow you to eat fast food or junk food in any quantity every day. Achieving a healthier lifestyle also means changing the way you eat to provide your body with healthy, beneficial nutrients that it can use.

This doesn't mean you'll need to cut out bread or buy the low-fat version of everything to lose weight, and it doesn't mean you need to get rid of fast food or junk food completely. The biggest part of eating better is being responsible about what and how much you're putting in your tank.

Portion Sizes and Servings

This is possibly one of the biggest issues we all face, sometimes without realizing it. We're about to tell you a saying that's not new, but that has a ton of truth to it: Your eyes *are* bigger than your stomach!

Piling food onto our plate without thinking about the portions we've got versus the actual serving size trains us to, as our moms and dads always insisted, clean our plate, even if there's too much on it.

How much you need to eat in a day depends on your metabolism, your level of exercise (how many calories you burn daily), your age, and several other factors. For many of us, though, moderate regular exercise coupled with occupying an office chair eight hours a day, five days per week, doesn't justify filling half a plate with mashed potatoes at dinner time.

So, look at the serving sizes on the boxes you buy, or look them up online. Actually measure your food out. If the box says one serving of rice is two-thirds of a cup, get out your measuring cup. Guesstimating what we think two-thirds of a cup looks like also gets us in trouble.

Counting Calories

Counting calories can be stressful, nor does it really need to be done actively with a calculator all the time. It's not necessarily a healthy mindset to rely on a calorie count app *before* you decide what you're "allowed" to have, and it should never be a locked gate standing in between you and foods you enjoy. You don't need to cut high-calorie foods off your list completely.

However, we do find that knowing the caloric count of foods versus your daily recommended caloric intake (which you can find online) is a helpful eye-opener. Recognizing where the bulk of your calories are coming from and why can help you to be more mindful overall of what you're eating and how it's affecting your body.

Knowing when food is high in calories, and using this knowledge to choose an appropriate portion size, sets you on a path toward wiser food choices.

It's Not All About the Fat

We're always hearing that if we want to lose weight, we need to reduce our fat intake. While this does carry some truth, certain fats are essential to the body and to our daily intake. It's knowing which fats to include and which fats to reduce that's key.

An avocado, for example, is not a low-fat food, but it's lauded as a superfood for a healthy diet. Why? This is because, although an avocado is 15% fat, these fats are mostly healthy monounsaturated fats that are good for your body.

Even saturated fats, which have long been vilified, are not as bad for you as you might think. Saturated fats are found in things like red meat and full-fat milk or cheese and are also beneficial to your body when in moderation. If you're responsible with keeping saturated fats at no more than 10% of your caloric intake, they're nothing to avoid.

Overconsumption of trans fats, on the other hand, found in margarine and fried foods, are responsible for more of our health issues. You don't need to cut them out completely, but they should be a "once in a while" thing.

You Don't Have to Give up Sugar

...But you should keep sugar in moderation, also. Sugar has addictive qualities, which is why we crave it.

If you're thinking that having a healthier lifestyle overall means you can never have ice cream, chocolate, soda, or cookies again, that's not the case.

It's all about portion size and control. Having dessert would mean having a serving of ice cream, not a pint of ice cream. You don't need to cut out soda completely, but you should limit it to one or two days a week. It's having one or more sodas every day that forms a dependency and gets us in trouble.

Make sugary foods your "sometimes" treat, and by all means, have a cookie or two...just don't sit down with the whole box.

Foods You Can Count On

Keeping all our most important food groups in mind, here are some examples of tried and true good go-to foods that can help transform your life and lead you toward your health goals.

Proteins

- Poultry – Turkey, Chicken, Duck
- Seafood – Salmon, Shrimp, Tilapia, Tuna, Sardines
- Meat – Beef, Pork
- Eggs
- Legumes – Beans (Black, Kidney, White, Garbanzo, etc.), Lentils

Carbs (Vegetables and Fruits)

- Broccoli
- Kale
- Spinach
- Zucchini
- Bell Pepper
- Squash
- Asparagus
- Brussels Sprouts
- Carrots

- Mushrooms
- Potatoes
- Sweet Potatoes and Yams
- Apples
- Bananas
- Oranges
- Kiwi
- Berries
- Pears
- Plums
- Peaches

Carbs (Wheat and Grains)

- Oatmeal
- Granola
- Quinoa
- Brown Rice
- Granola
- Whole wheat or multigrain bread.

Fats

- Seeds and Nuts – Almonds, Walnuts, Pistachios, Chia Seeds, Pumpkin Seeds.
- Nut Butters
- Olive Oil

Dairy (Fat and Protein)

- Milk – 1% to 2% milkfat.
- Cheese – Goat Cheese, Feta Cheese, Real Cheddar Cheese (not Kraft Singles).

- Yogurt

Applying Your Foods

We've got no doubt you've seen a list like we've given above many other places before. We also know that it's not enough just to know what foods are good for you, because most of us already know, generally, what they are. Now, we need to know how to apply these foods to our meal routine.

Building Nutrient Balance

Proteins, carbs, and healthy fats should all be present in your daily intake.

In general, it's recommended that carbs compose around 45% to 60% of your daily calories. Proteins should compose around 10% to 35% of your calories. And last but not least, fats should make up for 20% to 35% of your calories.

So, try to design meals for yourself, especially for breakfast and dinner, that incorporate all three groups.

A breakfast of a serving of yogurt (protein and fats), combined with a serving of granola or fresh fruit (carbs), and even a sprinkling of sunflower seeds (fats), composes a well-rounded breakfast.

A dinner of a serving of chicken breast (protein), a serving of asparagus (carbs), a serving of quinoa (carbs), and half an avocado (fats) will keep you fuller longer, give you the energy you need, and supply your body with useful nutrients.

Keep the Fat You Cook With in Mind

One tablespoon of any cooking fat, be it olive oil, vegetable oil, or butter, equates to 100 calories. And while cooking with olive oil is better for you than cooking with butter, going all-out with olive oil can add a lot of extra calories to your meal (oops!). So, try to measure out your cooking oils and try to reduce foods fried in a large amount of oil.

Don't Make Yourself Miserable

This may be the most useful piece of advice we can give, for a very good reason.

Cutting things completely out of your diet, like fats or carbs, or cutting out foods you enjoy, can result in vitamin and nutrient deficiency and trouble with lethargy, among other things.

Not only that, but cutting out every food you enjoy because someone insists that it's "bad" for you is what often causes "slingshot" diets, where we keep a diet up for an amount of time, then break it and over-eat the foods we were depriving ourselves of.

It's not healthy for your mind or your body and creates a vicious negative cycle. Yes, you need to be mindful of your intake, but that doesn't mean you can't have some beers with your friends on Fridays.

Structuring your diet into a list of "can have" and "can't have" often makes us miserable over time, leads to resentment and self-shaming when we indulge in the foods we've identified as "can't have."

Let go of the guilt associated with indulgence in food and drink typically associated as "bad for you." Understand that having a serving of ice cream now and again does not mean you've "failed." Our endeavors toward a healthier diet and overall life are a constant practice in self-control. Instead of thinking of a bowl of ice cream as "cheating," think of it as a treat, and develop your ability to control the portion and the frequency. The power to resist finishing the pint is in your hands!

Conclusion

Thank you very much for taking the time to read this book! Let's hope it inspired you to conquer your fitness goals and opened your eyes to new ways to work for a toned body.

If you're a beginner, you should now have an arsenal of exercises to work into your routine that is achievable for you and yet difficult enough to provide you with a challenge. If you're advanced, you should now have more exercises to add to your training regimen that put your body to work in ways you didn't know were possible.

The next step is to develop a schedule for yourself based on what you learned here. Identify the times during the day when you have a moment to work with your resistance bands and stick to them! Exercising itself is tough, but the toughest part is making it a regular part of your life. Your health and strength goals are important, so think of your exercise time as an essential activity to your day.

We also encourage you to keep track of your progress or to even share your progress with family and friends if you are so inclined. Seeing a positive difference in yourself across your fitness journey, as well as others seeing positive differences in you, can be very rewarding and provide you with extra motivation to keep pushing for your existing and new goals.

Finally, if you found this book useful in any way, a review on Amazon is always appreciated!